Principles and Practice Series

TOTAL INTRAVENOUS ANAESTHESIA

Principles and Practice Series

TOTAL INTRAVENOUS ANAESTHESIA

IAN SMITH BSc, MBBS, FRCA
Senior Lecturer in Anaesthesia,
Keele University, North Staffordshire Hospital,
Stoke-on-Trent, Staffordshire, UK

PAUL F WHITE PhD, MD, FANZCA
Professor and McDermott Chair of Anesthesiology,
University of Texas Southwestern Medical Center,
Dallas, Texas, USA

Principles and Practice in Anaesthesia Series edited by

C E W HAHN
University Lecturer in Anaesthetics,
Oxford University and Consultant in Clinical Measurement,
Oxford Radcliffe Hospital

and

A P ADAMS
Professor of Anaesthetics, University of London,
United Medical and Dental Schools of Guy's and St Thomas' Hospitals
and Honorary Consultant Anaesthetist, Guy's,
King's and St Thomas' Hospitals, London

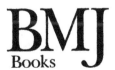

© BMJ Books 1998

BMJ Books is an imprint of the BMJ Publishing Group

All rights reserved. No part of this publication may be reproduced, stored in a retrieval system, or transmitted, in any form or by any means, electronic, mechanical, photocopying, recording and/or otherwise, without the prior written permission of the publishers.

First published in 1998
by BMJ Books, BMA House, Tavistock Square,
London WC1H 9JR

British Library Cataloguing in Publication Data

A catalogue record for this book is available
from the British Library

ISBN 0-7279-1191-0

Typeset by Apek Typesetters, Nailsea, Bristol

Contents

Glossary

ACTH	adrenocorticotrophic hormone
ADH	antidiuretic hormone
AIP	acute intermittent porphyria
BCDFE	2-bromo-2-chloro-1,1-difluroethylene (halothane break-down product)
BIS	bispectral index
BP	blood pressure
$C_{(t)}$	concentration at time t
C_0	initial drug concentration
CACI	computer assisted continuous infusion
cAMP	cyclic adenosine monophosphate
CBF	cerebral blood flow
Cl	clearance
$CMRO_2$	cerebral metabolic requirement for oxygen
CNS	central nervous system
CO_2	carbon dioxide
CPB	cardiopulmonary bypass
CPP	cerebral perfusion pressure
CSA	compressed spectral array (processed EEG)
CSF	cerebrospinal fluid
CT	computed tomography
C_T	target drug concentration
CVS	cardiovascular system
ECT	electroconvulsive therapy
EC_{50}	drug concentration at which the effect is half of maximum effect (sometimes called ED50)
ED_{50}	for a drug with a quantal (all or none) effect, this is the dose producing a response in 50% of a population. For a drug with a graduated response, it is the dose producing an effect which is half the maximum effect
ED_{90}	for a drug with a quantal (all or none) effect, this is the dose producing a response in 90% of a population. For a drug with a graduated response, it is the dose producing an effect which is 90% of the maximum effect
ED_{95}	for a drug with a quantal (all or none) effect, this is the dose producing a response in 95% of a population. For a drug

	with a graduated response, it is the dose producing an effect which is 95% of the maximum effect
EEG	electroncephalogram
E_{max}	maximum drug effect
EMLA	eutectic mixture of local anaesthetics (topical anaesthetic cream)
ETT	endotracheal tube
FiO$_2$	inspired oxygen fraction
FRI	fixed rate infusion
GABA	gamma amino butyric acid
HR	heart rate
5HT$_3$	5-hydroxytryptamine receptor (type 3)
Hz	hertz
IB	intermittent bolus doses
ICP	intracranial pressure
ICU	intensive care unit
IFT	isolated forearm technique
iv	intravenous
LEC	lower oesophageal (esophageal) contractility
LMA	laryngeal mask airway
LVEDP	left ventricular end diastolic pressure
MAC	minimum alveolar concentration
MAP	mean arterial blood pressure
MH	malignant hyperpyrexia
MRI	magnetic resonance imaging
N$_2$O	nitrous oxide
NLA	neurolept analgesia
NLAN	neurolept anaesthesia
NSAID	non-steroidal antiinflammatory drug
O$_2$	oxygen
PAP	pulmonary artery pressure
PCA	patient controlled analgesia
PCS	patient controlled sedation
PONV	postoperative nausea and vomiting
ppm	parts per million
PVR	pulmonary vascular resistance
RVSW	right ventricular stroke work
SEF	spectral edge frequency (processed EEG)
SpO$_2$	haemoglobin oxygen saturation
$T_{1/2}\gamma$	elimination half life
TCI	target controlled infusion
TFA	trifluroacetic acid
TIVA	total intravenous anaesthesia
TOF	train of four

Vd	volume of distribution
Vd_{ss}	volume of distribution at steady state
VEP	visual evoked potential
$V_{peak\ effect}$	the volume of distribution at peak drug effect
VRI	variable rate infusion
V_{ss}	volume of distribution at steady state

Preface

The original concept of total intravenous anaesthesia (TIVA) involved the use of a combination of intravenous sedative-hypnotic, analgesic, and muscle relaxant drugs to produce a state of general anaesthesia. However, the use of intravenous sedative-analgesic drugs in combination with local or regional anaesthetic techniques represents an increasingly popular form of intravenous anaesthesia. The latter technique is commonly referred to as a variant of monitored anaesthesia care (MAC).

Since the successful implementation of TIVA requires an understanding of basic pharmacokinetic and dynamic principles, this book provides an overview of the pharmacology of the major intravenous anaesthetic drug groups. In addition, the importance of drug interactions which can produce both synergistic and antagonistic effects is stressed. Finally, the roles of novel intravenous drug delivery (e.g. target controlled infusions (TCI)) and monitoring (e.g. EEG bispectral (BIS)) systems in intravenous anaesthesia are discussed.

The idea for this book on TIVA techniques grew out of a larger project on this topic. The recently published textbook *Intravenous Anesthesia* (Williams and Wilkins, Philadelphia) provides a comprehensive review of all the drugs and techniques used for producing an intravenous anaesthetic state. This book is intended to provide the anaesthesia and critical care trainee with an introduction to the basic concepts of intravenous anaesthesia by focusing on the role of TIVA. Although TIVA techniques have long been utilised for a wide variety of specialised procedures (e.g. cardiac and neurosurgical anaesthesia, electroconvulsive therapy (ECT)), the availability of the intravenous anaesthetic propofol has led to the more widespread use of TIVA for an increasing variety of surgical procedures.

With the availability of more rapid and shorter acting intravenous anaesthetic drugs, the ability to titrate these pharmacological agents to specific clinical endpoints has been improved. As improved techniques for delivering and monitoring intravenous anaesthetics are introduced into clinical practice, the use of TIVA techniques may eventually become as widespread as the inhaled (volatile) anaesthetics. Hopefully, this book will facilitate the education of anaesthesia practitioners regarding the use of intravenous anaesthetic techniques in their clinical practice.

Paul F. White PhD, MD, FANZCA
Dallas, Texas

1: Historical and scientific background of intravenous anaesthesia

Introduction

Although it is difficult to imagine the prospect of surgery without anaesthesia, it is sobering to recall that our specialty is only a little over 150 years old. Initially, anaesthesia was achieved by inhalation of gases and vapours and to this day, the instantly recognisable "cartoon" anaesthetist is always depicted with black rubber face mask and tubing. In reality, intravenous drugs have revolutionised the practice of modern anaesthesia. Most patients expect, and routinely receive, "an injection" to render them unconscious, while intravenous analgesics, muscle relaxants, and vasoactive drugs are regularly used during the maintenance of anaesthesia. Although it has been possible for many years to maintain an adequate anaesthetic using only intravenously administered drugs, most practitioners still use inhaled vapours and gases as maintenance agents in their everyday anaesthetic practice.

There are many reasons why inhaled agents still remain popular for the maintenance of anaesthesia, despite the almost universal use of intravenous induction agents. In part it is due to habit, while a lack of appropriate equipment, knowledge, and confidence also contributes to the relative unpopularity of intravenous anaesthesia. The aim of this book is to provide a broad and practical guide to intravenous anaesthesia, setting out the underlying scientific principles and examining the potential and real advantages (and disadvantages) of intravenous anaesthesia compared to inhalational techniques. Various intravenous anaesthetic techniques will be described, as will their utilisation in particular patient populations. The pharmacokinetic and pharmacodynamic properties of the various intravenous anaesthetic, analgesic, muscle relaxant, and adjuvant drugs will be discussed in some detail. This section will focus on those clinically useful drugs which are most commonly employed, but will also briefly summarise some of the new drugs which will become available in the near future.

It is not our intention for this book to be totally comprehensive. Neither was it intended that every statement should be referenced to the published literature, although the material is firmly based on scientific evidence. References are given to some of the more important or significant clinical studies, as well as to review articles where topics may be covered in greater depth. The remaining material has been synthesised from a variety of sources (including the author's personal experience). Many of the more recent facts have been extracted from a new and comprehensive textbook on intravenous anaesthesia,[1] to which we would happily refer those readers wishing to examine a particular topic in greater depth than that which is possible here.

History of total intravenous anaesthesia

Medicinal compounds were first injected soon after the circulation was described by Harvey in the 17th century. Interestingly, this achievement predates the invention of both the syringe and hollow needle, a bladder and quill being used for the first intravenous drug administrations. Although opium had been used for centuries and was also one of the first substances to be given intravenously, the idea of using intravenous opium for perioperative pain relief does not appear to have occurred until much later. The birth date of anaesthesia is accepted to be October 16th 1846 when ether was successfully demonstrated in public in Boston. Although one or two pioneers had actually achieved an anaesthetic state previous to this, they had also used inhaled agents. Ether anaesthesia was a major revelation and the technique spread rapidly around the world. As soon as the concept of anaesthesia had become established, however, dissatisfaction with some aspects of ether anaesthesia (especially the slow and unpleasant induction) led to a search for alternative agents. Although most of the early alternatives were also given by inhalation, iv agents began to be investigated a few years later. One of the first attempts to produce iv anaesthesia involved injection of chloral hydrate in the early 1870s, although a high mortality rate led to abandonment of the technique. Toxicity of the available compounds inhibited further developments until the next century, while inhaled anaesthesia continued unchallenged.

Enthusiasm for iv anaesthesia was revitalised in 1909 when hedonal was used successfully.[2] This was a derivative of urethane which had previously been used to treat insomnia. Hedonal was somewhat safer than previous iv anaesthetics, although it was relatively insoluble in water, making administration difficult, and was associated with a slow onset and recovery. The first barbiturate (somnifen) used for iv anaesthesia was introduced in 1921. A great variety of barbiturates were synthesised and much was learnt of their structure–activity relationships. The first short acting barbiturate (hexobarbione) was synthesised in 1932, and thiopentone, which had fewer excitatory side effects, was introduced in 1934. Thiopentone remains in use to this day, although its popularity has declined considerably since the introduction of propofol. Thiopentone is still considered by many to be the "gold standard", however, against which any new iv anaesthetic must be compared.

Although the barbiturates were a significant advance over previously available iv anaesthetics, they were associated with a number of problems. Many barbiturates had significant excitatory or convulsant effects, which prevented the employment of otherwise useful drugs. Most of the

---

Simplified chronology of iv anaesthesia

3rd century BC	Opium used for analgesia and recreation
16th century	Curare used as arrow poison
Mid 17th century	First medicines injected iv
1803	Morphine isolated from opium
1845	Hollow needle invented
1846	**Ether anaesthesia demonstrated**
1853	Syringe invented
1872	Chloral hydrate given iv
1909	Urethane derivative used for iv anaesthesia
1910	Concept of balanced anaesthesia
1921	First barbiturate introduced
1934	Thiopentone introduced
1939	Pethidine synthesised (first synthetic opioid)
1941	Pearl Harbor; iv anaesthesia described as "ideal method of euthanasia"
	Anaesthetic properties of steroids recognised
1942	Curare introduced
1950	Pharmacokinetics introduced to anaesthesia
1954	Artificial hibernation
1955	First benzodiazepine synthesised
	First anaesthetic steroid (hydroxydione)
1957	Methohexitone introduced
1959	Neurolept analgesia described
1960	Diazepam introduced
1965	Ketamine and propranidid introduced
1967	Fentanyl introduced
1969	High dose opioid anaesthesia proposed
1972	Althesin introduced
1974	Etomidate introduced
	Sufentanil synthesised
1976	Alfentanil synthesised
1979	Midazolam and minaxalone introduced
	Flumazenil synthesised
1980	Minaxalone withdrawn
1984	Propofol introduced
	Propranidid and Althesin withdrawn
1996	Remifentanil introduced
	TCI propofol commercially available

remaining barbiturates were associated with a prolonged duration of effect when given in large or multiple doses for maintenance of anaesthesia. The barbiturates also had significant cardiovascular depressant properties. These were exaggerated when large doses were given (without nitrous oxide [N$_2$O] or other adjuvants) as a sole anaesthetic or when used in association with hypovolaemia. The mass casualties from the attack on Pearl Harbor in 1941 roughly coincided with the peak of enthusiasm for "single agent" anaesthesia with barbiturates. Intravenous anaesthesia seemed ideal in the war or disaster setting. The drugs were easy to transport, being light and compactly packaged, and did not require particularly stringent storage requirements. Furthermore, they were non-flammable and non-explosive, a considerable advantage over ether and cyclopropane. Unfortunately, many deaths resulted from inadequate resuscitation of severely injured casualties and inappropriate doses of thiopentone and other barbiturates administered by poorly trained personnel. One contemporary report described intravenous anaesthesia as "an ideal method of euthanasia".[3] Although the effect of thiopentone on the number of casualties has probably been exaggerated, this event nevertheless impeded the development of iv anaesthesia.

A variety of non-barbiturates were developed, beginning in 1955 with the first steroid anaesthetic, hydroxydione. Unlike many other anaesthetic steroids, this drug was relatively stable in aqueous solution. However, it had a slow onset and a prolonged duration of action which, along with an unacceptably high incidence of thrombophlebitis, led to its early withdrawal. Several other steroid anaesthetics were evaluated, the most successful of which were the Althesin steroids alphaxalone and alphadolone, introduced in 1972 (chapter 3). Althesin was the most clinically useful steroid anaesthetic so far developed, with properties to rival those of propofol, introduced 12 years later. Problems with anaphylactic reactions caused by the solvent cremophor EL led to the withdrawal of Althesin and propranidid, another useful non-barbiturate anaesthetic, in 1984.

In the same year, propofol was launched in the United Kingdom. Propofol has since become the mainstay of iv anaesthesia, because of its predictably short duration of action which facilitates control of anaesthesia and rapid recovery, as well as its generally favourable side effect profile (chapter 3). Propofol almost suffered the same fate as Althesin and propranidid, initially being formulated in cremophor EL. Fortunately, the problems of this solvent were recognised and it was possible to reformulate propofol in a lipid emulsion prior to its clinical release. Similar attempts to reformulate the earlier anaesthetics have not been so successful.

A few other iv anaesthetics were introduced over the years which still retain a place today. Methohexitone, introduced in 1957, was widely used as a short lasting alternative to thiopentone until the availability of Althesin and subsequently propofol which had even shorter durations of effect.

Methohexitone is still used during electroconvulsive therapy (ECT) because of its predictable effect on seizure duration, but is little used elsewhere. Ketamine was introduced in 1965. When used on its own, hallucinations and emergence reactions were severe and significantly limited the acceptability of ketamine. Although these side effects have subsequently been modified by the coadministration of benzodiazepines, ketamine has never achieved great popularity and remains as a drug to be used under exceptional circumstances. Etomidate has also been available for over 20 years. Although it is associated with less cardiovascular depression than most other iv induction agents, it produces a number of other problems, including thrombophlebitis, nausea and vomiting and inhibition of steroid synthesis, all of which have limited its use (chapter 3). More recently, etomidate has been reformulated in a lipid solvent, which appears to reduce many of these problems. It is possible that etomidate may enjoy renewed popularity if these problems can be solved or reduced to an acceptable degree.

The first of the muscle relaxants, curare, was introduced into anaesthesia in 1942, having been used for a few years previously to reduce fractures resulting from convulsive therapy in psychiatry. In fact, curare was first used in surgery as early as 1912, but the report in a German journal was overlooked by other workers. Interestingly, the use of muscle relaxants in general anaesthesia predates by some years the routine use of mechanical, positive pressure ventilation. Early muscle relaxants were relatively non-specific, with a variety of side effects. Although a number of synthetic muscle relaxants were developed over the years, vecuronium (developed in 1980) was the first relatively specific non-depolarising muscle relaxant, associated with minimal side effects. Subsequently, a number of specific drugs of varying duration and rate of onset have been developed (chapter 3). Although muscle relaxants are not required for all operations, they are valuable adjuncts in many situations and it is now usually possible to select a drug with appropriate properties for most circumstances. The use of muscle relaxants does introduce problems, however. In particular, it removes useful early signs of inadequate anaesthesia and may increase the risk of intraoperative awareness (chapter 5).

From the early days of anaesthesia, it was frequently believed that an anaesthetic state should be achieved using a single agent, given in as large a dose as necessary to produce all of the desired effects. This practice was common in the early days of volatile anaesthetics and was repeated in the early attempts to use barbiturates for anaesthesia. In both cases, significant problems were encountered, with fatalities from profound respiratory and/ or cardiovascular depression. The concept of a balanced approach to anaesthesia was first proposed as long ago as 1910, with the idea of combining local infiltration analgesia with light general anaesthesia. The idea was further expanded in the 1920s to include premedication with regional and general anaesthesia. The more modern approach of N_2O, opioid analgesia, and hypnotic agent began to evolve in the 1940s and 1950s. Once more, there was a move back towards single agent anaesthesia in the late 1960s when the concept of high dose opioid "anaesthesia" was proposed for cardiac surgical procedures. Yet again, the technique proved disastrous, with a high incidence of muscle rigidity and intraoperative awareness. Today, most anaesthetics use a balanced approach with, at minimum, a hypnotic and an analgesic, commonly supplemented by N_2O. Another variant of the balanced anaesthetic approach is neurolept anaesthesia (chapter 2), which had its origins in the 1950s but evolved further in the late 1960s with the availability of fentanyl and droperidol. Although the technique had much to commend it in terms of safety relative to contemporary alternatives, it was also associated with a high incidence of unpleasant and undesirable side effects and has gradually been displaced from use by more modern techniques in developed countries.

Basic pharmacokinetics and pharmacodynamics

Use of intravenous agents to provide appropriate effects in the optimum time frame requires a basic knowledge of pharmacokinetic and pharmacodynamic principles. Pharmacokinetics describes the relationship between delivered dose and plasma concentration, popularly referred to as "what the body does to the drug". Pharmacodynamics describes the relationship between plasma concentration and clinical effect or "what the drug does to the body".

Basic pharmacokinetics

A fundamental pharmacokinetic principle is volume of distribution. If a known dose of drug is administered and its concentration in the plasma is subsequently measured, it is easy to calculate the volume into which the drug appears to have mixed (known as the volume of distribution) by dividing the drug dose by the plasma concentration. Mathematically, this is stated:

$$\text{Volume of distribution (Vd)} = \frac{\text{Amount of drug given}}{\text{Plasma concentration}}$$

The volume of distribution does not necessarily reflect the actual volume of plasma or other bodily tissues, but is simply a mathematical concept. For this reason it is often referred to as the apparent volume of distribution. Although the calculation assumes even distribution, this need not happen in practice. For example, a drug which extensively binds to tissues will have a lower plasma concentration for a given dose than a drug which remains largely in the plasma. As a result, the former drug will have a much larger volume of distribution than the latter.

Another important term is "clearance", which is the body's ability to remove drug from the blood or plasma. Clearance may occur by way of renal excretion, hepatic metabolism, and a variety of other means. It is often most useful to consider total body clearance, which is the combination of all these individual clearances. As clearance is expressed as the part of the volume of distribution from which drug is completely removed in a given time period, it has the units of flow, which are volume/time. Clearance is calculated from the decline in measured plasma concentration over time. Mathematically, this can be stated:

$$\text{Clearance (Cl)} = \frac{\text{Rate of drug removal}}{\text{Plasma concentration}}$$

As a result, the rate of drug removal depends on the plasma concentration of drug. For example, if the clearance of a drug is 1 l/min, 1 mg of drug will be cleared per minute if the plasma concentration is 1 mg/l, while 50 mg will be cleared for a plasma concentration of 50 mg/l and so on.

These concepts may be more easily visualised by using a hydraulic model involving a tank of water with a pipe at the bottom (fig 1.1). In this model, the volume of water corresponds to the amount of drug, the size of the pipe corresponds to the clearance, and the cross-sectional area of the tank corresponds to the volume of distribution. For a given amount of water, the larger the cross-sectional area of the tank, the lower the height of water. Using this simple model, the higher the level of water, the faster it will run out of the pipe, due to increasing water pressure. The "clearance" of water

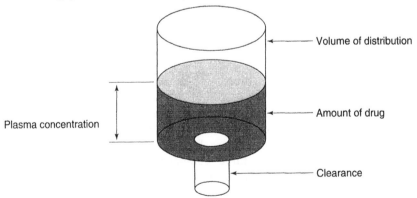

Fig 1.1 Simple hydraulic model representing the distribution of drug within the plasma. The cross-sectional area of the tank represents the volume of distribution, the volume of water represents the amount of drug, and its height corresponds to the plasma concentration. The clearance is determined by the size of the drainage pipe

(drug) is a first order process because it is directly proportional to pressure (concentration). In a first order process, drug concentration declines according to the following equation:

$$C(t) = C_0 \cdot e^{-kt}$$

where $C(t)$ is the concentration at time t, C_0 is the initial drug concentration, t is the time following its administration, e is the base of the natural logarithm, and k is the rate constant for elimination ($k = Cl/Vd$). The units of k are time^{-1} and the half life of this process is $0 \cdot 693/k$. If the concentration is plotted on a logarithmic scale, a straight line will be produced with slope of k and a y intercept of C_0, the initial drug concentration.

When drug is now supplied by a continuous infusion, the plasma concentration rises gradually until an equilibrium is achieved where the rate of drug administration is exactly balanced by drug elimination. At this point the plasma drug concentration will remain constant. Using just an infusion, the plasma concentration reaches half of its eventual level after one half life, 75% after two half lives, and 87·5% after three half lives. After five half lives, 97% of the final concentration has been reached and this is generally taken to be steady state. At steady state, the rate of flow out of the body (clearance) is equal to the rate of flow into the body (infusion rate). To achieve a desired (or target) concentration (C_T) with a continuous infusion will take a long time unless the drug has a very short half life. To reach this endpoint more rapidly, it is necessary to administer a bolus dose to achieve the target concentration, followed by an infusion in order to maintain it. The bolus dose is equal to the target concentration divided by the volume of distribution (C_T/Vd), while the infusion rate is equal to the target concentration times the clearance ($C_T \cdot Cl$). Traditional loading dose/ maintenance rate regimens such as these are useful for a variety of drugs in medicine.

The three compartment model

The discussion so far relates to drugs which are administered into, distributed within, and eliminated from a single compartment. In contrast, most drugs used in anaesthesia are better described by two or three compartment models. In a three compartment model, the drug is administered into and eliminated from a "central compartment", which is connected to two "peripheral compartments" (fig 1.2). Initially, the drug is only present in the central compartment. With time, however, it distributes into the two peripheral compartments. The peripheral compartment with which the plasma equilibrates more rapidly is (logically) termed the "rapid peripheral volume", sometimes referred to mathematically as V_2 (because the central compartment is V_1). By the same reasoning, the compartment with which equilibration occurs more slowly is known as the "slow peripheral volume" or V_3. The sum of all three compartment volumes is the volume of distribution at steady state, V_{ss}. Drug removal from the central volume is termed "central clearance", also known as metabolic or elimination clearance. Distribution of drug from the central to peripheral volumes also represents a form of clearance, "intercompartmental" or "distribution clearance". These are further subdivided into "rapid inter-compartmental clearance" and "slow intercompartmental clearance".

The volumes of the three compartment model do not relate to discrete anatomical sites but are simply mathematical constants derived from equations that describe the plasma drug concentrations over time. The central volume represents the space into which the drug is initially dissolved. This includes the blood, but also some tissues that have very high blood flow. It is possible to measure the central clearance with some accuracy, as it represents the sum of all processes which clear drug from the body (e.g. renal excretion, hepatic metabolism, enzymatic metabolism).

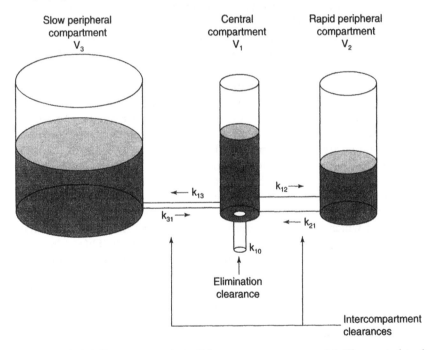

Fig 1.2 Hydraulic representation of three compartment model. The central tank represents the central compartment or volume (V_1), which equilibrates fairly rapidly (note large diameter connecting pipe) with the rapid peripheral compartment (V_2) and more slowly (note small diameter connecting pipe) with the slow peripheral compartment (V_3). Note that elimination (central clearance) occurs only from the central compartment. Microrate constants (k) for intercompartmental clearance are also shown

The intercompartmental clearances are influenced by blood flow and capillary permeability, but can be obtained from mathematical equations which describe the changes in the plasma concentration over time. In a three compartment model, the time course of the drug concentration can be described by a plasma concentration curve with three phases. The "rapid distribution phase" begins immediately after the bolus dose and is due to movement of drug from plasma to the rapidly equilibrating tissues. This is followed by a second "slow distribution phase" which is due to movement of drug into more slowly equilibrating tissues but also includes return of drug from the most rapidly equilibrating tissues back into the plasma. The "terminal phase" (which is almost a straight line on a semilogarithmic plot) represents drug elimination from the body, as well as drug returning to the plasma from both distribution volumes. This returning drug tends to reduce the rate at which the plasma concentration decreases. Although the terminal phase is often called the "elimination phase", this is somewhat misleading as elimination is occurring during all three phases.

The movement of drug between compartments can also be described by a series of "microrate constants", abbreviated as k. For example, k_{12} defines the rate of drug transfer from compartment 1 to compartment 2, while k_{21} defines the rate of transfer in the opposite direction. To completely describe a three compartment model requires five rate constants: one for the transfer of drug from the central compartment to the rapid peripheral compartment, another for transfer in the opposite direction, a second pair governing transfer between the central and slow peripheral compartments, and a fifth for elimination (fig 1.2). Although the differential equations derived from these constants are too complex to be of practical use in the clinical administration of iv anaesthetics, they can be used to programme computers to simulate drug behaviour or to deliver approximately constant plasma drug concentrations (see chapter 5).

The three compartment model can also be described in terms of three half lives, of which two are distribution half lives and the third a terminal half life which is also often referred to as the "elimination half life". The half life of a drug is often referred to in drug related literature and it is invariably the terminal half life which is mentioned, rather than the distribution half lives. As the terminal half life only refers to the final phase of the concentration–time curve, it bears little relationship to the decrease in plasma concentration after a bolus dose or a continuous infusion of drug and therefore does not predict clinical duration of effect.[4] The terminal (or elimination) half life is always greater than the time it will actually take for plasma concentrations of drug to decrease by 50% after the end of drug administration. Furthermore, the time for the plasma concentration to decrease is highly dependent upon the preceding duration of drug administration, with blood levels decreasing more slowly (sometimes much more slowly) after long infusions compared to bolus doses.

10

Predicting decline in plasma concentration

The rate of decrease in plasma (and brain) concentration is important as it determines, amongst other things, awakening from an anaesthetic. As the terminal half life is a poor measure of this decline for drugs described by multicompartmental pharmacokinetics and the interactions of the different clearances, volumes, and diffusion constants are complex, a simple measure is needed to predict clinical recovery. In 1992, Hughes and colleagues introduced the term "context sensitive half time".[5] The "half time" is the time required for a 50% decrease in plasma concentration following infusions of varying duration, with the "context" being the preceding duration of infusion at which a steady state drug concentration was maintained. By definition, then, the context sensitive half time is not a single value but is better represented as a continuous curve of half time against infusion duration. For illustration, curves of the context sensitive half times of a series of opioid analgesics are shown in fig 1.3.[6] An alternative approach is to list half times for bolus administration as well as for infusions of short, intermediate, and long duration.

Pharmacodynamic considerations

Pharmacodynamics is the relationship between drug concentration and effect. For most drugs, this response is in the shape of a sigmoidal curve (fig 1.4). At zero concentration, there will be no effect. There will also be a concentration which produces the maximum effect (E_{max}). Once E_{max} is

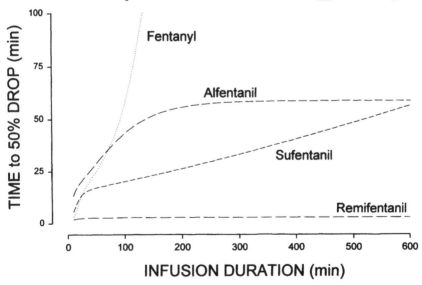

Fig 1.3 Simulated times required for a 50% decrease in plasma concentration after variable length continuous infusions (context sensitive half time) of fentanyl, alfentanil, sufentanil, and remifentanil. Reproduced with permission[6]

11

reached (perhaps because all the receptors are fully occupied), further increases in drug concentrations have no additional effect. It is also possible to determine the EC_{50}, the concentration (strictly speaking, the effect site concentration, see below) at which the effect is half E_{max}. The EC_{50} is used as an index of drug potency when comparing drugs with similar effects. Less potent drugs require a higher concentration in order to achieve a similar effect to a lower concentration of a more potent drug. Note that potency refers to the relationship between concentration and effect; the dose–effect relationship is also influenced by pharmacokinetic factors. Potency is also not synonymous with efficacy. E_{max} is the measure of a drug's efficacy. A low potency drug can achieve the same E_{max} with a sufficiently large dose, but a drug with a low E_{max} is always less effective at producing a particular effect, no matter how high its concentration.

The sigmoidal relationship described defines a continuous response to a

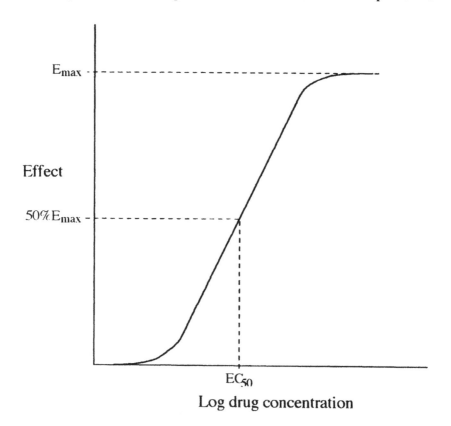

Fig 1.4 The effect of a drug at a variety of escalating doses. E_{max} represents the maximal achievable effect and EC_{50} the drug concentration which produces an effect which is 50% of E_{max}

drug in an average individual, but can also be used to characterise the probability of reaching a quantal effect (response/no response) in a particular population. An example would be the anaesthetic concentration required to prevent response to various stimuli (e.g. intubation, skin incision, skin closure) in 50% of patients. For a continuous response, the steepness of the sigmoid curve reflects the ease with which a drug can be titrated between no effect and maximum effect (fig 1.5). For a quantal effect, the steepness of the curve is related to the amount of variability in the patient population. Drugs with steep curves will have little variability between patients in concentration and effect. These relationships can be used to define a therapeutic window to suggest an initial choice of the optimal drug concentration. It is also important to know how a drug's concentration relates to its toxic effects as well as to its therapeutic effect. This information helps to define the upper limits of the drug's therapeutic window.

Another important aspect is the diffusion of drug from the plasma to its site of action. Although plasma concentrations peak almost instantly, the

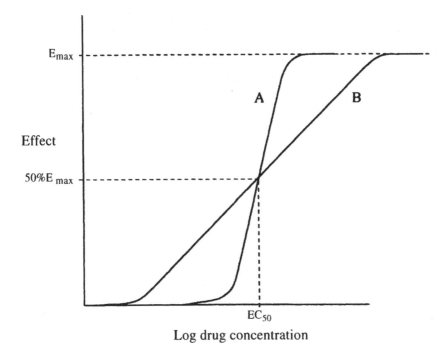

Log drug concentration

Fig 1.5   Drugs A and B both produce a similar maximal effect (E_{max}) and have a similar EC_{50}. Drug A has a much steeper dose–response curve compared to drug B, such that there is a narrower range between the dose which produces no effect and that which produces maximal effect. Consequently, drug A will be more difficult to titrate to a desired clinical effect than drug B

plasma is usually not the site of drug action, only a means of transport to that site. The biological effects of drugs occur at the "biophase" (or "effect compartment") which may be a variety of biological sites, including membranes and receptors. The biophase is small and inaccessible, so the drug concentration there cannot be measured. If a measure of drug effect (e.g. neuromuscular junction monitor, electroencephalogram) exists, however, it is possible to characterise the time course of a drug's effect and therefore its rate of flow into and out of the biophase. A microrate constant describing the transfer of drug out of the central compartment (biophase) and into the central compartment can be defined. This is termed k_{e0} (although logically it should really be k_{e1}). This allows an effect compartment to be added to the pharmacodynamic model in order to describe more accurately the onset of drug effect (fig 1.6). Because the effect compartment is so small, it has no influence on the remainder of a drug's pharmacokinetics.

The time to peak effect site concentration (and therefore to peak effect) after a drug bolus is a function of both pharmacokinetic factors and k_{e0}. Where the plasma concentration declines very rapidly following a bolus dose, the effect-site concentration will peak rapidly, regardless of the k_{e0} value. For drugs whose concentration declines more slowly following a bolus injection, however, the time to peak effect site concentration is determined predominantly by the k_{e0}. k_{e0} is rapid for thiopentone, propofol, and alfentanil, intermediate for fentanyl and sufentanil, and most muscle relaxants, and slow for morphine and ketorolac.

While the effect site is equilibrating with plasma, the plasma concentra-

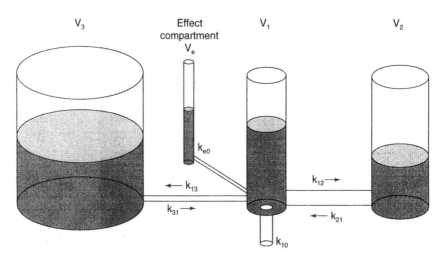

Fig 1.6   Hydraulic representation of three compartment model incorporating the effect compartment. Note the small size of the effect compartment and the microrate constant (k_{e0}) for transfer to the central compartment

tion continues to decline, due mainly to drug redistribution. As drugs always diffuse down concentration gradients, the peak effect site concentration of a slowly equilibrating drug will be lower than that of a rapidly equilibrating one as the plasma concentration at the time of peak effect site concentration will also be lower. In order to achieve a comparable peak effect, a larger dose of a slowly equilibrating drug will be needed relative to a rapidly equilibrating one. This will result in a larger amount of drug reaching peripheral tissues, which will delay recovery and may also increase side effects.

For the one compartment model, it was easy to determine the dose necessary to produce a desired plasma concentration using the formula: dose $= C_T \cdot Vd$. For a three compartment model with an effect site, however, this formula is difficult to use because we do not know which volume to use for Vd. If the volume of the central compartment (V_1) is used, the calculated dose will be too small, as some of the drug is redistributed or eliminated before reaching the effect site. Alternatively, using the volume at steady state (Vdss) results in too large a dose, as it normally takes many hours for drugs to spread equally throughout the compartments. If, however, the ratio between the initial plasma concentration and the plasma concentration at the time of peak effect is known, it is possible to calculate the volume into which the bolus dose appears to have distributed at the time that the peak effect is achieved. This calculated volume is referred to as the "volume of distribution at peak effect" and referred to by the term $V_{peak\ effect}$. This volume is entirely theoretical as the plasma concentration changes from its initial value to that at the time of peak effect by a combination of redistribution and elimination. Nevertheless, the term $V_{peak\ effect}$ is adequate for the purpose of calculating the necessary bolus dose.

Maintaining a constant plasma concentration with a three compartment model is again more complex than the simple formula $Cl \cdot C_T$ used in the one compartment model. To maintain a constant effect site concentration, an infusion should be started as soon as the peak effect is achieved. At the time of peak effect there will be no concentration gradient between the plasma and the effect site, so if that plasma concentration can be maintained, so will be that at the effect site. In order to achieve this, the infusion rate must match the rate of flow of drug out of the central compartment to the rapid distribution volume (V_2) and to the slow distribution volume (V_3) as well as elimination from the body. These calculations are too complex to be useful for manual drug delivery schemes but can readily be performed by computer. Computer driven drug infusions can either be used to achieve a relatively constant plasma (or effect site) concentration or the system can be made to increase or decrease the effect site concentration, depending upon the clinical response. A pharmacokinetic based infusion device is now commercially available for propofol (Diprifusor), and it is likely that a number of devices suitable for use with a range of anaesthetic drugs will become available over the next few years (see chapter 5).

Summary

Although anaesthesia has a long history, many of the significant developments have been made in recent years. Most of the drugs currently in use have been developed in the last 20 years, many more recently than that. As our understanding of structure activity relationships improves, it is possible to design drugs with desirable properties. Much has been achieved in this respect with benzodiazepines, opioids, and muscle relaxants. As we learn more of the mechanism of action of iv hypnotics, we can expect newer drug developments there also.

Improved understanding of pharmacokinetic principles has led to an improved ability to predict plasma concentrations (and resulting effects) following drug administration. This allows the best choice of drug for a particular effect and also allows us to use existing drugs more logically in order to achieve an appropriate effect rapidly and maintain it at a chosen level for as long as required. Optimal drug delivery should also avoid administration of more drug than necessary, reducing side effects and ensuring the fastest possible recovery at the end of drug administration. Understanding which pharmacokinetic parameters are important allows us to predict more accurately the behaviour of new drugs under various circumstances.

When planning bolus doses or infusion rates based on pharmacokinetic parameters, it should be remembered that these relate to healthy adults of average weight and build. Variations in these factors, as well as the effect of underlying disease processes, will influence both pharmacokinetics and pharmacodynamics. It is therefore necessary to adjust the dosing regimen to each individual patient's needs. It is not yet possible to mathematically correct for physiological and pathological variations, allowing suitably modified formulae to be used. The optimal effect is still achieved by observing the clinical effect (and side effects) and adjusting the dosing strategy accordingly. We are now moving towards the use of computers, programmed with pharmacokinetic data, to deliver iv anaesthetics. Already these devices appear promising, yet in comparison to the history of inhaled anaesthesia, we are still only a little beyond the ether stage. We have made a lot of progress to date, but we still have some way to go.

1 White PF, ed. *Intravenous anesthesia*. Baltimore: Williams and Wilkins, 1997.
2 Kissin I, Wright AG. The introduction of hedonal: a Russian contribution to intravenous anesthesia. *Anesthesiology* 1988;**69**:242–5.
3 Halford FJ. A critique of intravenous anesthesia in war surgery. *Anesthesiology* 1943;4:67–9.
4 Shafer SL, Varvel JR. Pharmacokinetics, pharmacodynamics, and rational opioid selection.

Anesthesiology 1991;74:53–63.

5 Hughes MA, Glass PSA, Jacobs JR. Context-sensitive half-time in multicompartment pharmacokinetic models for intravenous anesthetic drugs. *Anesthesiology* 1992;76:334–41.

6 Egan TD, Lemmens HJM, Fiset P, *et al.* The pharmacokinetics of the new short-acting opioid remifentanil (G187084B) in healthy adult male volunteers. *Anesthesiology* 1993;79:881–92.

2: Types of intravenous anaesthesia

Introduction

In 1990, Mallon and Edelist[1] made the prediction that "There is no doubt that total intravenous anaesthesia (TIVA) is a concept whose time has come...". Some eight years later, most practitioners are still awaiting the "arrival" of TIVA as a routine clinical practice. Although TIVA techniques have become popular for cardiac and neurosurgical procedures, "routine" general anaesthesia is most commonly performed using a combination of intravenous and inhaled anaesthetic drugs. In this chapter, the use of intravenous anaesthetic drugs as part of a variety of general anaesthetic techniques will be described.

Balanced anaesthesia

In the early days of anaesthesia, most patients received only a single anaesthetic drug (e.g. ether, nitrous oxide or chloroform). Relatively little of these drugs needed to be given for superficial surgical procedures, but when more intense analgesia or more profound muscle relaxation was required, it was necessary to administer high concentrations of the chosen drug to provide sufficiently "deep" anaesthesia. In modern clinical practice, it is usual to provide loss of consciousness, analgesia, muscle relaxation, and autonomic stability by the simultaneous administration of several specific drugs. When this is achieved using a combination of intravenous and inhaled anaesthetics, it is referred to as "balanced anaesthesia".

This concept of combining various drugs was probably first suggested by George Washington Crile of Cleveland, Ohio, who developed the concept of anoci-association. Crile advocated the use of light anaesthesia to prevent the effects of auditory, visual, and olfactory stimuli, while local anaesthetics were used to obtund the pain of surgery. The term "balanced anaesthesia" was first used by John Lundy in 1926. It was suggested that the use of small amounts of several drugs would avoid the side effects caused by a large dose of a single drug, thereby increasing patient safety and improving the flexibility of anaesthesia. Lundy used a combination of premedication, regional, and general anaesthesia to provide unconsciousness and pain relief in his "balanced" technique. This practice of combining several drugs to administer anaesthesia may be safer than the use of only one or two drugs. Evidence for the apparent safety of this balanced approach comes from a recent survey of 100 000 anaesthetics which revealed that the relative odds of death within seven days of surgery were 2.9 times greater when one or two anaesthetic drugs were used compared to the use of three or more.[2]

When thiopentone was first introduced, it was used as a sole anaesthetic. By 1938, it was being used with nitrous oxide, which permitted a reduction in the barbiturate dose yet provided superior anaesthesia to that obtained with thiopentone alone. Since patients receiving this combination were simultaneously recovering from low doses of two drugs, rather than a large dose of one, return of consciousness was significantly faster than when thiopentone was used without nitrous oxide (N_2O). To this date, N_2O is still used as an analgesic component of most anaesthetic techniques, irrespective of whether the primary anaesthetic is an iv agent or a volatile anaesthetic.

The practice of balanced anaesthesia advanced considerably when Griffith and Johnson introduced the muscle relaxant curare in 1942.[3] Anaesthetists could now achieve adequate muscle relaxation without having to administer large amounts of general anaesthetics. When Grays and Rees introduced the concept of the "triad of anaesthesia" in 1952, they defined its three essential components as narcosis, analgesia, and muscle relaxation.[4] This triad was expanded into a tetrad by Woodbridge in 1957, who added abolition of autonomic reflexes as a fourth essential aspect.[5] The supplemental analgesia provided by N_2O was generally insufficient to reliably prevent signs of sympathetic stimulation during surgery. In order to achieve all the components of "balanced anaesthesia", pethidine (meperidine) was introduced to supplement thiopentone, d-tubocurarine and N_2O anaesthesia.

Subsequently, a great many opioid analgesics have been developed and incorporated into balanced anaesthesia. Similarly, there have been improvements in both hypnotic agents and muscle relaxants. Adjuvant drugs have also been developed, specifically to control the autonomic responses to surgery. Despite improvements in each of the individual components of the anaesthetic tetrad, a balanced approach has remained the most effective. For example, after the development of the potent opioids (e.g. fentanyl, sufentanil, and alfentanil), it was suggested that anaesthesia for cardiac surgery was best performed with large doses of opioids given with oxygen and a muscle relaxant. The result was a high incidence of chest wall rigidity, intraoperative awareness and prolonged postoperative respiratory depression necessitating an extended period of assisted ventilation in the ICU. Although moderately high doses of opioids are still used in critically ill patients to achieve haemodynamic stability, a more balanced approach allows excellent intraoperative conditions and can hasten recovery.

19

Neurolept and dissociative anaesthesia

Neurolept anaesthesia originated in an attempt to alleviate the high mortality associated with the use of inappropriate doses of thiopentone in severely hypovolaemic patients. Henry Laborit, a French navy surgeon, observed what he described as "postaggressive disease" in his postoperative patients. Assuming this to be a stress response, he tried to attenuate it by using phenergan to reduce the sympathetic overactivity of the "neurovegetative" system. Phenergan has antiadrenergic, antihistaminic, and antiemetic properties, but neither induces unconsciousness nor provides any analgesia. It was therefore combined with pethidine (meperidine) for analgesia and chlorpromazine, a "neurolept" agent, in order to obtain more detachment from the surrounding environment. Laborit named this new mixture a "lytic cocktail".

From the original neurolept mixture, a variety of other neurolept compounds (phenothiazine derivatives, butyrophenones, benzamides, and thioxanthene) have been developed and used clinically in various combinations. Although inappropriate dosing and misuse of neurolept agents caused serious complications in the early days of neurolept techniques, no deaths occurred during the first ten-year period, in contrast to the many fatalities associated with inhalation anaesthetics of this time. The original neurolept technique was further modified by the addition of hypothermia to produce "artificial hibernation", during which hypothermia and hypometabolism provided a degree of cellular protection. Early advances in both cardiothoracic and neurosurgery were dependent on these anaesthetic techniques.

Pethidine, as used in the original lytic cocktail, is of limited analgesic potency. When fentanyl was synthesised with substantially greater analgesia potency and a higher safety margin, it was combined with the neurolept agents (haloperidol and droperidol) into "neuroleptanalgesia" (NLA). A commercial preparation of fentanyl 50 µg/ml and droperidol 2·5 mg/ml was produced under the trade name of Innovar™. This was also administered with diazepam as a coinduction agent which reduced the dose of Innovar and improved haemodynamic stability. This technique was known as neurolept anaesthesia (NLAN).

Neurolept drugs

Neurolepsis was first observed after the administration of haloperidol. A variety of vegetative, psychic, and motor functions are suppressed in this syndrome. At modest doses, emetic symptoms are prevented, while larger doses induce catalepsy. Although droperidol is associated with fewer side effects than many other neurolept drugs, it can still produce dyskinesia, restlessness, hyperactivity, chills and shivering, dysphoria with inner anxiety, hallucinations, and loss of body image. Similar effects are produced even more commonly after other butyrophenones. In contrast, the phenothiazines cause orthostatic hypotension, hypothermia, and sympatholytic activity. It is primarily because of these frequent and unpleasant side effects that neurolept anaesthesia/analgesia has become much less popular in recent years.

Pharmacokinetics

Droperidol has a duration of clinical effect of 3–6 h, its elimination half life is about 100 min, total body clearance is 14 ml/kg/min, and the apparent volume of distribution is 2 l/kg. Droperidol is highly lipid soluble and is extensively taken up by a variety of tissues. As droperidol has a slower onset and a longer duration of effect than fentanyl, separate administration of these two drugs is more appropriate than the use of a fixed combination such as that present in Innovar. Ideally, a loading dose of droperidol should be administered first, after which fentanyl should be administered in small increments (25–50 µg) or by infusion. Alternatively, one of the newer synthetic opioids (e.g. alfentanil, sufentanil, remifentanil) may be used in place of fentanyl.

Practical aspects of NLA and NLAN

The traditional fentanyl-droperidol (Innovar) NLAN technique is still being practised in many parts of the world. In the United Kingdom, the USA, and other parts of western Europe, however, the technique has become much less common. This is due in part to the fixed ratio of fentanyl and droperidol in Innovar. While the dysphoria resulting from this mixture was thought likely to discourage the illicit use of the opioid analgesic, it is also disadvantageous for patients. The relative overdose of droperidol consequent upon the use of this fixed ratio combination resulted in many adverse haemodynamic and psychological sequelae.

Although a few enthusiasts still administer droperidol and fentanyl separately for NLA (for example, "dope and drope" is still practised at the University of Texas Southwestern Medical Center in Dallas), the technique has largely been superseded by the improved intravenous (and volatile) hypnotic agents now available. Droperidol in low doses (1·25 mg) is still frequently used as a prophylactic antiemetic, although postoperative dysphoria is still observed even after such small doses.[6] Advocates of NLA and NLAN claim that a major advantage of these techniques is avoidance of postoperative nausea and vomiting and that NLAN is therefore appropriate for procedures where these side effects are especially undesirable (e.g. eye surgery, ENT procedures). The availability of propofol, however, with its direct antiemetic properties, as well as increased use of non-opioid forms of analgesia (e.g. NSAIDs, local anaesthesia) provide a better alternative. In addition, where prophylactic antiemetics are required (e.g. "high risk" patients or procedures), the $5HT_3$ antagonists are more effective and have fewer side effects. In cardiac surgery, NLAN combines a rapid induction of unconsciousness with cardiovascular stability, moderate α-adrenergic blockade, good perioperative analgesia, and minimal depression of airway reflexes. Traditional neurolept anaesthesia certainly compared well with thiopentone–halothane–N_2O anaesthesia in reducing the incidence of hypotension and hypertension and at the time, NLAN was a significant advance in cardiac anaesthesia. It has now largely been displaced, however, by the combination of moderate to high dose opioids with infusions of propofol (or even small doses of the newer volatile anaesthetics).

A variant of NLAN is the anaesthetic state produced by ketamine, an unusual form of catalepsy, termed "dissociative anaesthesia". Because of the adverse side effects associated with ketamine (see chapter 3), it soon became common to coadminister ketamine with diazepam. This so-called ataract analgesia became another new form of NLAN. Combinations of ketamine with benzodiazepines have also been used for cardiac anaesthesia where they produced haemodynamic conditions as good as or better than those possible with alternative anaesthetics available at the time.

Total intravenous anaesthesia (TIVA)

As its name implies, total intravenous anaesthesia is a technique involving the induction and maintenance of anaesthesia with intravenous (iv) drugs alone. Each separate component of anaesthesia (e.g. unconsciousness, analgesia, amnesia, control of the autonomic nervous system, muscle relaxation) is provided and regulated by selecting specific iv agents. It differs from balanced anaesthesia in that, in addition to volatile agents, N_2O is also avoided.

In common with balanced anaesthesia, TIVA is claimed to avoid the hazards associated with volatile anaesthetic agents (table 2.1). In addition, TIVA is useful for preexisting conditions or surgical procedures in which N_2O may be contraindicated or where its administration may be difficult

Table 2.1   Possible hazards of volatile anaesthetics

Cardiovascular   Cardiovascular depression (enflurane > isoflurane > halothane)
   Cardiovascular stimulation (desflurane)
   Possibility of coronary steal (isoflurane)
CNS   Cerebral vasodilation
     Epileptic activity (enflurane)
Respiratory   Respiratory irritant (desflurane > isoflurane > enflurane)
   Prevent pulmonary hypoxic vasoconstriction
Toxicity   Hepatotoxicity (halothane > enflurane > isoflurane > desflurane)
   Nephrotoxicity (methoxyflurane ?enflurane)
   Malignant hyperpyrexia
   Operating room pollution

Table 2.2   Possible hazards of nitrous oxide (N_2O)

Cardiovascular	Cardiovascular depression
Gastrointestinal	Probably increases nausea and vomiting
Pressure effects	Air embolism (including microemboli following CPB)
Pneumothorax, lung cysts, and bullae	
Middle ear surgery	
Bowel obstruction or prolonged bowel surgery	
Pneumencephalography (rarely performed now)	
Toxicity	Diffusion hypoxia
Bone marrow dysfunction with chronic exposure	
Possible foetal abnormalities with trace quantities	
Miscellaneous	Supports combustion (airway laser surgery)
Prevents administration of high FiO_2	
Logistical problems (hot climate, field situation)	

(table 2.2). By eliminating N_2O, it is possible to administer a much higher concentration of oxygen. This may be especially beneficial during one-lung anaesthesia and in other patients at risk of hypoxaemia or ischaemia. There may be other situations (e.g. bronchoscopy, high frequency jet ventilation) where it is technically easier to ventilate the patient's lungs using oxygen or air/oxygen mixtures while ensuring adequate anaesthesia and analgesia with a TIVA technique. It is also claimed that TIVA can decrease the incidence of postoperative nausea and vomiting (PONV), primarily by the avoidance of N_2O. However, in order to compensate for the omission of N_2O, analgesia must be provided by alternative means, usually involving opioids, which may themselves induce PONV. In addition, larger doses of intravenous hypnotic agents are also required compared to balanced anaesthesia techniques, which may result in delayed recovery unless very short acting drugs are used and their dosages adjusted carefully. The requirements for increased amounts of iv drugs will also substantially increase direct costs, although it is hoped that these will be offset by faster recovery and a shorter postoperative stay and/or a reduced requirement for drugs and other measures required to treat PONV and other side effects.

The means of drug administration is important in order to achieve an adequate anaesthetic state and will be discussed in greater detail later (see chapter 5). Intermittent bolus injections will result in high peak plasma concentrations of drug, resulting in excessive anaesthesia and possible side effects, alternating with troughs associated with inadequate anaesthesia and the possibility of awareness. However, if boluses are administered at too short an interval, drug accumulation may occur, which may delay recovery. More precise control may be achieved by administering short acting drugs by continuous infusion.[7] Relatively complex administration regimens are required, involving a bolus dose (or loading infusion) to rapidly achieve an adequate blood concentration of drug, followed by a diminishing infusion rate to compensate for drug redistribution while maintaining an effective concentration at the drug's site of action. In addition to these manoeuvres which are required because of the drug's pharmacokinetic properties, it may also be necessary to titrate the rate of drug administration to compensate for changes in the level of surgical stimulation.

Since TIVA involves the administration of both hypnotic and analgesic drugs, a variety of infusion strategies are possible. The infusion rate of the hypnotic drug may be held constant for the majority of the surgical procedure while the analgesic drug infusion is altered in response to variations in stimulus intensity and patient response. Alternatively, the analgesic infusion may be maintained and the hypnotic varied or both infusions may be adjusted independently.

It would appear logical to fix the opioid at an analgesic effect site concentration and adjust the hypnotic infusion. However, the intensity of the nociceptive (surgical) stimulus varies with time and setting the analgesic level sufficiently high to obtund responses to the most severe level of pain may result in relative overdosage of opioid and delay the return of spontaneous ventilation at the end of the operation. As the required level of unconsciousness does not change during the course of surgery, in contrast to the required level of analgesia, periods of "inadequate" anaesthesia may be better treated by increasing the plasma analgesic concentration. When using alfentanil and propofol as part of a TIVA technique, Monk and colleagues found that acute hypertensive responses could be treated significantly more rapidly with alterations in alfentanil administration (6 min) compared to propofol (10 min).[8] Maintaining a constant hypnotic infusion and adjusting the analgesic also resulted in earlier postoperative awakening.[8] Consideration should also be given to the pharmacokinetic properties of the individual drugs when deciding which infusion to alter. It would seem logical to titrate the drug with the most rapid onset and offset of action while the relatively longer lasting component is maintained at a steady state concentration just above the minimally effective level at its site of action. The availability of remifentanil, with its extremely short context sensitive half time of three minutes, should make it substantially easier to adjust the analgesic component of a TIVA regimen.

Where both the hypnotic and analgesic drug infusions are to be adjusted, the opioid infusion rate should be based on sympathetic activity and/or the expected intensity of the surgical stimulation. Adjustments in the hypnotic drug infusion rate should be made in response to patient movements or other clinical signs of inadequate anaesthesia. However, these clinical signs may be masked whenever large doses of muscle relaxants are used, making this strategy less suitable under these circumstances. Intraoperative awareness remains a major concern with TIVA and is one reason for the slow growth in popularity of this technique.

There is currently no accepted and reliable "depth of anaesthesia" monitor. Instead, the practitioner has to rely on clinical signs of adequate anaesthesia, of which the most reliable seem to be alterations in muscle tone and the pattern of respiration.[9] When muscle relaxants and controlled ventilation are used, these signs are lost and alternative endpoints are needed. Changes in blood pressure are a less reliable guide to the depth of anaesthesia with intravenous agents compared to inhalational anaesthetics,[10] while autonomic nervous system signs are unreliable when potent opioids or adrenergic blocking agents have been administered. Furthermore, many drugs used during anaesthesia directly interfere with autonomic responses independent of their anaesthetic effect(s).

Prevention of awareness relies on administering doses of opioids appropriate to the expected level of nociception and maintaining an effective level of hypnosis. Awareness is more likely when plasma concentrations are fluctuating widely. Unfortunately, the dose–response relationship for consciousness/unconsciousness is not known for most intravenous drugs. For propofol, however, blood concentrations of $3\cdot3$–$5\cdot4$ µg/ml are likely to prevent recall. If signs of light anaesthesia are observed, anaesthesia may be deepened rapidly by a bolus dose of propofol. It may require several minutes of inadequate anaesthesia before the patient is sufficiently aware for postoperative recall to occur, allowing adequate time for prevention provided that the anaesthetist remains vigilant. In addition, benzodiazepines may be used to prevent recall as they impair both explicit and implicit memory.[11]

Pharmacodynamics relevant to TIVA

Central nervous system (CNS) effects

With the exception of ketamine, all the intravenous drugs are cerebral vasoconstrictors. The iv hypnotics also depress cerebral metabolism and have little effect on cerebrovascular autoregulation or reactivity of the cerebrovascular system to CO_2. As a result, intracranial pressure will be unchanged or reduced, producing less swelling of the brain and better operating conditions. The improved oxygen supply and demand ratio achieved with TIVA may be especially beneficial in cerebral trauma or ischaemia.

Cardiovascular system (CVS) effects

TIVA has the ability to provide optimal haemodynamic control, although each component may have specific and dose related haemodynamic effects, which may be additive or synergistic if several drugs are administered together. Etomidate and the opioid analgesics probably cause the least cardiovascular depression and the reduction in systemic vascular resistance caused by the benzodiazepines is also generally relatively minor. The barbiturates cause a rather greater reduction in blood pressure, stroke volume, and systemic vascular resistance, while propofol has even greater effects because of vasodilation accompanied by a degree of negative inotropism. Despite these apparently adverse CVS effects, the myocardial oxygen supply and demand ratio is usually better maintained with TIVA than is the case with volatile agents, making these techniques a better choice to avoid myocardial ischaemia in patients with coronary artery disease or hypertension.

Respiratory system effects

Most iv anaesthetics produce dose dependent changes in tidal volume, respiratory rate, and expired minute volume. Unlike the volatile anaesthetics, however, several of the iv analgesics and hypnotics do not impair the pulmonary hypoxic vasoconstrictive reflex, which may permit better compensation for ventilation–perfusion mismatch. TIVA may be especially beneficial for maintaining anaesthesia while 100% O_2 is delivered (e.g. one-lung anaesthesia, severe pulmonary disease) or where gas delivery may be difficult (e.g. jet ventilation).

Miscellaneous effects

Intravenous anaesthetics appear to maintain adequate levels of hepatic and renal perfusion. There is no evidence of anaesthetic agent specific hepatotoxicity (which has been reported with halothane, enflurane, isoflurane, and desflurane) or nephrotoxicity (which occurred relatively frequently after methoxyflurane and is also a potential problem following enflurane). None of the iv anaesthetics serve to trigger malignant hyperpyrexia and several agents are also safe in porphyria.

Summary

In its broadest sense, balanced anaesthesia means the use of different drugs to provide each separate component of the anaesthetic tetrad. In this context, the term encompasses neurolept techniques, as well as TIVA, in which each component is provided by an intravenously administered drug. In more common usage, however, a balanced approach in the context of intravenous anaesthesia is taken to mean the use of N_2O as an analgesic supplement with all other components being supplied by iv drugs, while TIVA excludes the use of N_2O.

The modern concepts of balanced and total intravenous anaesthesia have evolved from the early experience with NLA and NLAN techniques. At the time, NLA and NLAN offered significant advantages over the other available options. Neurolept and dissociative anaesthetic techniques have always been associated with a high incidence of perioperative side effects. These side effects were an acceptable alternative to the high mortality associated with high dose barbiturate anaesthesia but with improvements in anaesthetic drugs, administration techniques, and patient selection, they served to limit the clinical acceptance of NLA and NLAN techniques.

Droperidol still maintains a place in the prophylaxis of postoperative nausea and vomiting, but at much lower doses than those used in neurolept techniques. Even with these reduced doses, side effects remain problematic and newer antiemetic drugs are beginning to displace droperidol. The introduction of ketamine and dissociative anaesthesia added a variant to NLAN which still maintains a small place today. The use of ketamine is, however, limited to a few unusual circumstances where its unique properties offer particular advantages over the available alternatives. In less developed societies where modern drugs may be unavailable and where skilled anaesthetists may be uncommon, NLAN (and especially dissociative anaesthesia) may still have a major place as a safe anaesthetic technique, albeit with many side effects.

TIVA is able to avoid a number of hazards and potential problems associated with volatile anaesthetics and N_2O. The technique allows all the essential components of anaesthesia to be delivered, using specific drugs, yet leaves the airway unencumbered for oxygenation and CO_2 removal. Because the iv drugs are generally more specific compared to volatile anaesthetics, the individual components of anaesthesia (e.g. hypnosis, analgesia, muscle relaxation, autonomic control) can be provided in degrees appropriate to the circumstances, with the potential to reduce adverse effects. The need to administer several drugs concurrently does allow for the development of drug interactions, however, and an understanding of the behaviour of drugs given alone and in various combinations is necessary for safe practice.

Because the duration of effect of iv drugs is dependent on redistribution and metabolism, however, a thorough knowledge of pharmacokinetic principles is essential in order to ensure optimal drug selection and dosage regimen. Pharmacokinetic modelling has been extremely useful in improving our understanding of how plasma concentrations decline following varying durations of drug administration. Improvements in drug development have resulted in agents with significantly shorter durations of effect (e.g. remifentanil) which make titration to effect much easier and also reduce the likelihood of an undesirably prolonged postoperative effect. It is likely that the future will see even more highly specific and shortlived iv anaesthetic and analgesic drugs, making TIVA an even more attractive proposition.

1 Mallon JS, Edelist G. Total intravenous anesthesia (editorial). *Can J Anaesth* 1990;37:279–81.
2 Cohen MM, Duncan PG, Tate RB. Does anesthesia contribute to operative mortality? *JAMA* 1988;260:2859–63.
3 Griffith HR, Johnson GE. The use of curare in general anesthesia. *Anesthesiology* 1942;3:418–20.
4 Gray TC, Rees GJ. The role of apnoea in general anesthesia. *Br J Anaesth* 1952;2:891–2.
5 Woodbridge PD. Changing concepts concerning depth of anesthesia. *Anesthesiology* 1957;18:536–50.
6 Melnick B, Sawyer R, Karambelkar D, Phitayakprn P, Uy NT. Delayed side effects of

3: Pharmacokinetics and pharmacodynamics of drugs used in total intravenous anaesthesia

Introduction

The availability of rapid and shorter acting intravenous anaesthetic, analgesic, and muscle relaxant drugs has facilitated the use of intravenous anaesthetic techniques in routine clinical practice. The ability to utilise a combination of highly specific pharmacologic agents to achieve precise clinical endpoints should further improve the practice of intravenous anaesthesia in the future. This chapter will review the pharmacokinetic and pharmacodynamic properties of the currently available sedative-hypnotic, opioid and non-opioid analgesic, muscle relaxant, and adjuvant drugs when used during intravenous anaesthesia.

Sedative-hypnotics

Propofol

Propofol was introduced into clinical practice in the late 1980s and has since become the most commonly used hypnotic component of iv anaesthesia. Although propofol was initially popular in day case anaesthesia, it is now frequently used for cardiac, neurosurgical, and paediatric anaesthesia, as well as for conscious sedation and sedation on the ICU. Anaesthesia is induced smoothly and rapidly and is associated with minimal side effects. Its clinical duration of action is acceptably short which permits a rapid recovery at the end of anaesthesia but also facilitates control of the depth of anaesthesia during the maintenance period by allowing rapid responses to changes in the delivered concentration.

Studies on the molecular mechanism of propofol's effects on the central nervous system (CNS) would suggest that, as with other CNS depressants (e.g. barbiturates, etomidate), propofol activates the $GABA_A$ receptor–

Table 3.1 Major pharmacokinetic parameters for the iv hypnotics

Drug	Protein binding (%)	V_C (l/kg)	V_{dss} (l/kg)	Clearance (ml/kg/min)
Propofol	98	0·1–0·4	2–12	20–28
Ketamine (racemic)	12	0·3–1·4	1·4–6·0	14–20
S(+) ketamine	-	0·4	-	30
Etomidate	65	0·15	2·5–4·5	18
Thiopentone	83	0·5	2·5	3·4
Methohexitone	73	0·35	2·2	10·9
Midazolam	96	0·17	1·1	6–10

V_C Volume of central compartment; V_{dss} Volume of distribution at steady state

chloride ionophore complex. At clinically relevant concentrations, propofol increases chloride conductance. However, at high concentrations of propofol desensitization of the $GABA_A$ receptor results in suppression of the inhibitory system.

Pharmacokinetics

The major pharmacokinetic values for propofol are shown in comparison to other iv hypnotic agents in table 3.1. Propofol is extensively (up to 98%) bound to plasma proteins. The pharmacokinetics of propofol are described by a typical three compartment model. The volume of the central compartment is quoted as 0·1–0·4 l/kg and the Vd_{ss} ranges from 2 to 12 l/kg. The short clinical duration of effect of propofol is due to both redistribution and rapid metabolic clearance. Following an initial bolus of propofol, plasma levels decline rapidly due mainly to redistribution of propofol from the brain and other highly perfused tissues into less well perfused sites (e.g. muscle). Although the initial distribution clearance of propofol is quite rapid (3–4 l/kg/min) it is no faster than thiopentone. However, subsequent metabolic clearance of propofol occurs at a rate which is approximately ten times faster than that of thiopentone and which exceeds hepatic blood flow, suggesting that propofol may be metabolised in extrahepatic sites. This suggestion is supported by the detection of metabolites when propofol is given during the anhepatic phase of orthotopic liver transplantation.

The elimination half life $(T_{1/2}\gamma)$ of propofol is long, yet recovery from its clinical effects is rapid, even after prolonged administration. The reason for this apparent discrepancy is that since propofol has a large steady state volume of distribution, it extensively redistributes into muscle, fat, and other poorly perfused tissues. These sites have a very large capacity, although they equilibrate with the central compartment only very slowly. As a result, the concentration in the central compartment will still be much higher than in these peripheral compartments, even at the end of a prolonged propofol infusion, so that redistribution will continue to occur after drug delivery stops. The concentration in the central compartment will rapidly decline, both from metabolism (elimination) and from continuing redistribution, until it is below that required for hypnosis (or deep sedation), permitting rapid awakening. When the concentration in the central compartment eventually becomes lower than that of the highly lipophilic tissue compartments (e.g. fat), propofol will begin to move back into the central compartment. However, this transfer occurs very slowly and propofol concentrations in the central compartment remain sub-therapeutic. Thus, the complete elimination of propofol from the body may take many hours or even days (as indicated by the long $T_{1/2}\gamma$ value), but has minimal effect on clinical recovery. Propofol has a context sensitive half time of less than 25 min following infusions lasting up to three hours and the half time is still only 50 min following prolonged infusions. If the propofol infusion is titrated to effect, so that the plasma propofol concentration has to decline by only 10–20% to permit awakening, recovery is very rapid.

As with the barbiturates, the elderly have a reduced dose requirement for propofol, due to a smaller central compartment and reduced clearance. In children, the volume of propofol's central compartment is larger on a per kg body weight basis than in adults and the clearance is also higher. Therefore, children will require a larger induction dose and an increased maintenance infusion rate (per kg body weight) than adults.

The clinical duration of effect of propofol does not appear to be greatly affected by obesity, moderate hepatic or renal dysfunction. Although propofol metabolites accumulate in patients with renal failure, the lack of differences in emergence times would suggest that these metabolites lack clinically significant effects. Since considerable interpatient variability exists in both healthy and sick patients, careful titration of the propofol dose to effect will minimise adverse effects such as hypotension, while permitting a rapid recovery from its central effects. For patients weighing 60–90 kg, a "standard" dose infusion regimen is a useful starting point. As part of a balanced or TIVA technique, infusion rates of 75–300 μg/kg/min are usually required, while adequate sedation can be maintained with infusion rates of 25–100 μg/kg/min (fig 3.1). It has become possible to define "target" plasma concentrations for hypnosis (2–6 μg/ml) and sedation (0·5–1·5 μg/ml) during a variety of clinical conditions (fig 3.2).

Pharmacodynamics

The effects of propofol on a variety of organ systems are summarised in comparison to other iv hypnotics in table 3.2.

CNS effects

Considerable interest has been shown in the use of propofol for maintenance of neurosurgical anaesthesia because a rapid recovery profile would facilitate an earlier postoperative assessment of CNS function. Propofol infusions can be used as an alternative to the volatile anaesthetic agents, which all have the ability to cause cerebrovascular dilation and thereby increase intracranial pressure (ICP). In contrast to the volatile anaesthetics, propofol is associated with cerebral vasoconstriction, decreased cerebral blood flow (CBF), and reduced cerebral metabolic rate for oxygen ($CMRO_2$). Although most studies have found a reduction in ICP following induction of anaesthesia with propofol, the associated decrease in mean arterial blood pressure (MAP) usually leads to a decreased cerebral perfusion pressure (CPP). It would appear that the autoregulatory capacity of the cerebral circulation remains intact during propofol anaesthesia and the response of the cerebrovascular system to changes in CO_2 tension is also preserved.

Although there are reports of involuntary movements and "convulsions" following propofol administration, several workers have confirmed the absence of seizure activity or epileptiform activity by EEG recording during involuntary movements with propofol. It is more likely that these excitatory events result from preferential depression of subcortical areas. Propofol does not produce seizure-like activity, even in patients with complex partial epilepsy, and has been successfully used to treat status epilepticus.[1] Excitatory events (e.g. myoclonus, tremor, and dystonic posturing) during induction of anaesthesia appear to be less prominent with propofol than

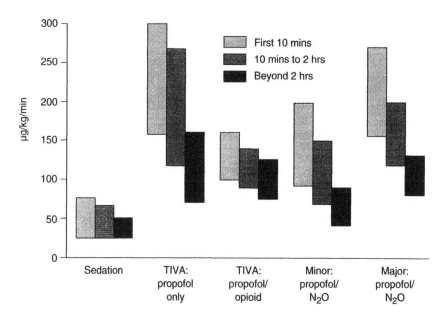

Fig 3.1 Recommended propofol infusion regimens to achieve satisfactory conditions for sedation, total intravenous anaesthesia (TIVA) with and without supplemental opioid analgesics and nitrous oxide supplemented anaesthesia for minor and major surgical procedures. Reproduced with permission[62]

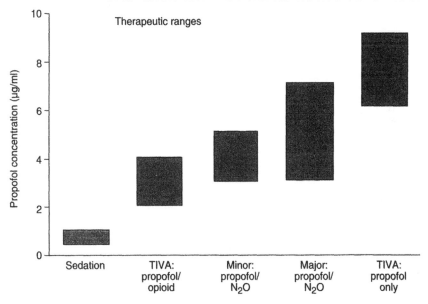

Fig 3.2   Therapeutic plasma propofol concentrations required for a variety of anaesthetic applications. Reproduced with permission[62]

with etomidate, thiopentone or methohexitone.[2]

CVS effects   Propofol reduces the systemic blood pressure more during induction of anaesthesia compared to alternative induction agents,[3] predominantly by way of peripheral vasodilation. The degree of hypotension produced is unlikely to be of clinical significance to healthy patients and can be reduced to some extent by careful and slow administration, augmented by adequate preoperative hydration. Propofol should be used with caution in patients with preexisting cardiac disease, however.

Propofol is becoming popular in cardiac anaesthesia as a supplement to high dose opioid techniques to improve haemodynamic stability, reduce intraoperative awareness, and improve the rate of recovery. Even the use of small doses of propofol (0·5 mg/kg) in combination with alfentanil (50 μg/ kg) results in hypotension following induction of anaesthesia.[4] Similar effects were observed with propofol 1 mg/kg and fentanyl 6 μg/kg, although no ECG evidence of myocardial ischaemia was noted during the periods of hypotension.[5] In comparison to alternative anaesthetic induction agents, propofol produces a greater degree of hypotension as a result of decreased venous tone and reductions in total peripheral resistance. In addition, in common with other hypnotics, there is an interaction with opioid analgesics which exacerbates these hypotensive effects.

The desire to avoid hypotension on induction, while maintaining haemodynamic stability during laryngoscopy, tracheal intubation, and

33

Table 3.2 Major pharmacodynamic properties of the iv hypnotics

Drug	Cardiovascular effects	Respiratory effects	Central nervous system effects	Other effects	Malignant hyperpyrexia	Porphyria
Propofol	↓↓↓MAP Vasodilation	Bronchodilator	↓CBF ↓CMRO$_2$ ↓ICP ↓CPP	Antiemetic Fast recovery Pain on injection	Safe	Safe
Ketamine (racemic)	↑MAP & HR Direct myocardial depressant	Minimal depression Excellent bronchodilator	↑CBF ↑CMRO$_2$ ↑ICP ↓CPP	Excellent analgesic Emergence phenomena	Safe	Safe
S(+) ketamine	As racemic ketamine	As racemic ketamine	As racemic ketamine	Improved emergence	Safe	Safe
Etomidate	↓MAP ↑HR Vasodilation	Minimal ventilatory depression	↓CBF ↓CMRO$_2$ ↓ICP ↔CPP	Inhibits steroidogenesis PONV Injection pain	Safe	Safe
Thiopentone	↓↓MAP ↑HR Vasodilation	Ventilatory depressant	↓CBF ↓CMRO$_2$ ↓ICP ↑CPP	Slow recovery Irritant to extravascular tissues	Safe	Unsafe
Methohexitone	↓↓MAP ↑↑HR Vasodilation	Ventilatory depressant	↓CBF ↓CMRO$_2$ ↓ICP ↑CPP Proconvulsant	Less irritant to tissues Faster recovery than thiopentone	Safe	Unsafe
Midazolam	↓MAP Vasodilation	Minimal ventilatory depression	↓CBF ↓CMRO$_2$ ↓ICP ↔CPP	Slow induction Useful as premed or coinduction	Safe	Unsafe

MAP Mean arterial pressure; HR Heart rate; CBF Cerebral blood flow; CMRO$_2$ Cerebral metabolic rate for oxygen; ICP Intracranial pressure; CPP Cerebral perfusion pressure sternotomy, led to the use of other sedative-opioid combinations for induction of anaesthesia followed by a propofol infusion for maintenance of anaesthesia. For example, following an opioid induction, a two stage propofol infusion produced comparable haemodynamic changes and a reduced requirement for vasodilator therapy compared to maintenance with enflurane.[6] In patients with decreased left ventricular function, an opioid induction (with sufentanil 5 µg/kg) followed by a variable rate propofol infusion (50–200 µg/kg/min) produced satisfactory control of haemodynamic variables, a decreased requirement for vasopressor medication, and less biochemical evidence of myocardial ischaemia compared to a sufentanil-enflurane group.[7] Propofol-opioid combinations have also been shown to produce more hypotension but less hypertension than opioid-midazolam combinations, with no differences in perioperative ischaemia or myocardial contractility.

The use of propofol for maintenance of cardiac anaesthesia is associated with a more rapid emergence from anaesthesia and earlier extubation compared to high dose fentanyl, enhancing the ability to "fast track" cardiac surgery patients and reduce their stay in the intensive care unit. For example, use of a propofol infusion (67–100 µg/kg/min) for maintenance of anaesthesia allowed haemodynamically stable patients to be weaned from ventilatory support as soon as consciousness returned, allowing a median time to extubation of two hours (with only 2·5% of patients requiring continuing ventilatory support at 24 h) compared to a median time to extubation of seven hours in a comparable group anaesthetised with an opioid based technique.[8]

Miscellaneous effects Propofol has a direct bronchodilating effect on bronchial smooth muscle (analogous to its relaxant effects on vascular smooth muscle). The potency of propofol in inhibiting adrenal steroidogenesis is 1500 times less than that of etomidate.[9] There is no evidence of a clinically significant impairment of steroidogenesis with propofol.[10] When used for electroconvulsive therapy (ECT), propofol consistently results in a shortened duration of seizure activity compared to thiopentone and methohexitone. Even so, the efficacy of ECT appears similar in patients anaesthetised with either propofol or methohexitone, despite shortened seizure duration in the propofol group. In addition, propofol is more effective than methohexitone in attenuating the rise in blood pressure and heart rate immediately after ECT which may offer protection against myocardial infarction, a not uncommon complication of ECT. Recovery following ECT appears to be more dependent on the duration of the seizure than the type of hypnotic administered and is not significantly shortened with propofol compared to methohexitone, however.[11]

Propofol based anaesthetics have been safely used for providing anaesthesia to patients susceptible to malignant hyperpyrexia (MH) as well as for muscle biopsy procedures in patients being tested for MH susceptibility. Propofol is safe in MH susceptible patients and does not affect the sensitivity of *in vitro* contracture testing.[12] Propofol has also been used safely in patients with a history of acute intermittent porphyria (AIP).

A major beneficial effect of propofol is its direct antiemetic activity,[13] which may be mediated via antagonism of the dopamine D_2 receptor.[14] Compared to volatile agents, the use of propofol for general anaesthesia is associated with less postoperative nausea and vomiting and/or decreased requirements for antiemetic medication.[15] Similar findings have been found when using propofol as an alternative to other intravenous induction or maintenance agents. The antiemetic effects of propofol are confirmed by its ability to treat nausea and vomiting when infused in subhypnotic doses; 10–20 mg of propofol successfully treated 81% of patients with PONV in the recovery room, compared to 35% of those given a lipid emulsion.[16] The antiemetic effects of propofol are shortlived, however, with six of the 21 patients experiencing a relapse within 30 min after receiving propofol. A subhypnotic dose (10 mg) of propofol also appears to protect against itching after intrathecal opioids and is equally effective to naloxone 2 µg/kg but with a lower incidence of postoperative pain.

A major problem with propofol administration is pain on injection, which occurs in 28–90% of patients. Although the mechanism responsible for the propofol induced venous pain is unknown, it has been suggested that it may be due to activation of the kinin cascade system. The pain is a function of propofol itself, rather than its formulation.[17] Pain on injection can be reduced by using large veins, by cooling propofol, and by dilution of propofol with either 5% glucose solution or 10% Intralipid. The most effective measure, however, is the addition of local anaesthetics (e.g. lignocaine 1–2%). The reduction in pain from the addition of lignocaine to propofol is dose related and up to 40 mg of lignocaine may be required. Lignocaine appears equally effective when mixed with the propofol or when given as a "pretreatment" dose. When a mixture is used, the lignocaine and propofol should be freshly mixed and used within 30 min, otherwise a significant fraction of the lignocaine will have entered the lipid phase and resulted in a decline in the free concentration. Although pain on injection is common with propofol, unlike diazepam and etomidate, this is not associated with phlebitis. Propofol also appears to be relatively harmless when inadvertently injected intraarterially or into the extravascular tissues.

In summary, propofol has become a commonly used intravenous hypnotic because of its rapid recovery and relatively beneficial side effect profile. Rapid recovery facilitates titration of dose to effect to optimise drug delivery and is also associated with rapid awakening after sedative doses, brief procedures, and even more prolonged administration. The antiemetic effects of propofol are advantageous in a variety of clinical circumstances and propofol is also a useful "universal" anaesthetic which can be used in "problem patients" (e.g. malignant hyperpyrexia, porphyria). Although propofol causes hypotension, this is seldom detrimental with cautious administration. The other major disadvantage, pain on injection, can be reduced significantly by lignocaine. To date, propofol has the best balance of clinical properties of all iv hypnotics. Although alternative agents may have distinct advantages in specific circumstances, they are inferior to propofol for the majority of patients and procedures.

Ketamine and its isomers

Ketamine, a phencyclidine derivative, was synthesised in 1963 and first used in humans in 1965. Ketamine produces a unique state of "dissociative anaesthesia",[18] in which the patient is in a cataleptic trancelike state (often with their eyes open), disconnected from their surroundings, accompanied by profound analgesia.

Ketamine hydrochloride is a water soluble white crystalline salt. Commercial preparations of ketamine are available as clear, colourless solutions which are stable at room temperature with a pH between 3·5 and 5·5. Commercial ketamine is a racemic mixture of two optically active isomers, S(+) ketamine and R(−) ketamine.[19]

Pharmacokinetics

The major pharmacokinetic values for ketamine are shown in comparison to other iv hypnotic agents in table 3.1. Ketamine has a low degree of plasma protein binding and is highly lipid soluble, leading to extensive distribution throughout the body, with apparent distribution volumes of 100–400 l. Ketamine has a large central volume of distribution (20–100 l) and a total body clearance of 1000–1600 ml/min. The terminal half life value ($T_{1/2}\beta$) is 2·5–3·0 h. Children have higher clearance rates, smaller volumes of distribution, and shorter elimination half life values compared to adults. The bioavailability of orally administered ketamine is low (<20%) due to first pass metabolism, although 93% is available following intramuscular injection.[20] The maximum plasma concentration is reached within five minutes of intramuscular delivery, while an iv bolus dose of ketamine (2 mg/kg) induces unconsciousness within 20–60 s, with emergence occurring 10–15 min later. As with other iv induction agents, recovery from an induction dose of ketamine is mainly by redistribution from the brain to poorly vascularised tissues.

Hepatic microsomal enzymes degrade ketamine into a number of metabolites, of which norketamine (N-demethylated ketamine) is the most important. Norketamine appears in the plasma 2–3 min after ketamine administration and reaches its peak level in 30 min. It is pharmacologically active with an anaesthetic and analgesic potency which is 3–10 times less than that of ketamine. Following further degradation, most ketamine metabolites are excreted in the urine. Coadministration of ketamine with benzodiazepines (or barbiturates) may prolong the terminal half life of ketamine, while diazepam competitively inhibits N-demethylation of ketamine, decreasing its hepatic clearance.

Pharmacodynamics

The effects of ketamine on a variety of organ systems are summarised in comparison to other iv hypnotics in table 3.2.

CNS effects   Ketamine initially produces a loss of EEG α activity combined with decreased amplitude and a variable effect on frequency followed by persistent rhythmic θ activity (4–6 Hz) at increased amplitude and finally intermittent high amplitude polymorphic δ activity (0·5–2 Hz).[21] Ketamine depresses some regions of the neocortex and subcortical structures (e.g. thalamus), while activating other parts of the limbic system (e.g. hippocampus), in contrast to other iv anaesthetics which cause more widespread CNS depression. This suggests that ketamine causes a functional dissociation between the limbic and thalamoneocortical systems. Hypnotic doses of ketamine also flatten visually evoked potentials (VEP) and alter acoustic evoked responses.

Ketamine is known to increase ICP, with greater changes occurring after intravenous administration compared to intramuscular injection. Transient increases of 1–60 mmHg have been observed in patients with intracranial pathology following an induction dose of ketamine. Increases in ICP have also been observed in healthy volunteers, although these are of lesser magnitude than in patients with abnormal intracranial compliance. The increase in ICP can be reduced by prior administration of sedatives and is unlikely to be of any clinical significance in healthy patients. Ketamine increases ICP by way of increased cerebral blood flow secondary to decreased cerebral vascular resistance. As the increase in ICP is usually greater than the corresponding increase in systemic arterial pressure, CPP will be reduced and ketamine should probably be avoided in patients with intracranial pathology or abnormal cerebral perfusion.

Despite conflicting reports regarding its epileptogenic properties, ketamine is less likely than natural sleep to activate epileptic discharges in patients with a history of focal or generalised epilepsy. Indeed, ketamine has potent anticonvulsant effects against generalised tonic-clonic seizures in animals.

CVS effects   In contrast to other iv induction agents, ketamine causes significant increases in HR, MAP, and plasma catecholamines. These circulatory effects of ketamine are caused by central sympathetic stimulation[22] and may be advantageous in patients with hypovolaemia or massive haemorrhage. Ketamine also causes a direct depressant effect on the myocardium following large bolus doses (>1.5 mg/kg) or rapid injection (<30 s). In most circumstances, this effect is more than compensated for by the sympathetic stimulation, although it may be problematic in the critically ill. Sympathetically mediated vasoconstriction also compensates for the direct vascular smooth muscle dilation produced by ketamine with the net effect being a minimal change in SVR. Ketamine increases coronary blood flow, although this may be insufficient to meet the increased metabolic demands of the heart caused by tachycardia and hypertension. Ketamine is contraindicated in patients with reduced right ventricular reserve as it increases pulmonary vascular resistance (PVR), pulmonary arterial pressure (PAP), and right ventricular stroke work (RVSW). During one-lung anaesthesia, ketamine maintains the hypoxic pulmonary vasoconstrictor response.

Respiratory system effects Ketamine causes minimal respiratory depression at usual induction doses. Respiratory depression can be produced, however, by the rapid injection of large doses of ketamine (>2 mg/kg) and is exacerbated by premedication with benzodiazepines. In contrast to other iv anaesthetics, ketamine is more likely to maintain normal functional residual capacity, minute ventilation, tidal volume, and the intercostal muscle contribution to ventilatory function. It produces a useful bronchodilating effect in asthmatic patients, which appears to be due to a direct effect on bronchial smooth muscle.

Ketamine increases salivary and tracheobronchial secretions and administration of an antisialogogue (e.g. glycopyrrolate 0.1–0.2 mg) has been recommended. As pharyngeal and laryngeal airway reflexes are usually well maintained, patients may be capable of maintaining an intact airway and swallowing during ketamine anaesthesia. Although aspiration is less likely with ketamine compared to other general anaesthetics, attention should still be given to protecting the airway of patients "at risk" of pulmonary aspiration.

Miscellaneous effects Ketamine increases uterine tone and the intensity of uterine contractions at anaesthetic doses (1–2 mg/kg); analgesic doses (0.2–0.4 mg/kg) have no discernible effects. Ketamine can be used for induction of anaesthesia for obstetric emergencies in order to maintain blood pressure and uterine contractility in the presence of acute haemorrhage while allowing the administration of 100% oxygen.

Ketamine's effect on IOP is similar to thiopentone and etomidate. It has been used safely in patients with acute intermittent porphyria, myopathies, and malignant hyperpyrexia.

Emergence phenomena

When ketamine is administered alone, emergence from anaesthesia is associated with dreams (pleasant and unpleasant), visual disturbances, hallucinations, illusions, "weird trips", floating sensations, alterations in mood, and delirium. These emergence reactions (especially hallucinations) can occur in up to 90% of patients but are more common in adults, females, habitual dreamers, and those with a previous history of psychological problems. Flashbacks, lasting several weeks, can occasionally occur following ketamine anaesthesia. These side effects are unaffected by covering the eyes or allowing patients to recover in a dark, quiet room. Atropine and other centrally active vagolytic drugs increase the incidence of psychotomimetic side effects. Droperidol is effective in reducing the cardiostimulant effects of ketamine, but does not reduce its psychotomimetic effects.[23] The psychotomimetic effects of ketamine can be reduced by a variety of sedatives, and currently the benzodiazepines provide the most practical and complete protection against both circulatory and psychotomimetic side effects.

Clinical uses of ketamine

The clinical usefulness of ketamine has been limited because of its cardiovascular and psychomimetic side effects, which persist to some extent even when ketamine is given with other sedative-hypnotic drugs (e.g. midazolam, propofol). Ketamine has become a valuable drug in specific clinical situations, however (table 3.3). Ketamine is ideal for use in wars and civilian disasters. The option of intramuscular delivery combined with relative preservation of airway reflexes makes ketamine the anaesthetic of choice where the patient is inaccessible (e.g. trapped casualties). The profound analgesic effects of ketamine are also useful during brief painful procedures (e.g. burn dressing changes, bone marrow biopsies, dural puncture, and removal of chest drains in children).

Because of its cardiostimulatory properties, ketamine is not ideal as a sole agent in patients with cardiac disease but may be more suitable when used with benzodiazepines. When high dose diazepam was used to prevent the ketamine induced increase in the rate-pressure product, adequate anaesthetic conditions with minimal cardiorespiratory effects were obtained during cardiac anaesthesia.[24] Compared to sufentanil, ketamine maintained a stable cardiac index and heart rate, but with increased wall tension in patients with severe cardiomyopathy undergoing cardiac transplantation.[25] When used to supplement fentanyl induced anaesthesia, ketamine causes less cardiovascular depression compared to other commonly used sedative hypnotics (e.g. thiopentone, etomidate). It also produces more prolonged postoperative analgesia following thoracic surgery compared to fentanyl.

Ketamine has been considered the drug of choice in patients with cardiac tamponade or constrictive pericarditis, because it maintains sympathetic

Table 3.3   Clinical uses of ketamine in the practice of anaesthesia

---

Induction (or maintenance) of anaesthesia in high risk patients
  Shock or cardiovascular instability
  Severe dehydration
  Bronchospasm
  Severe anaemia
  One-lung anaesthesia
Obstetric practice
  Induction of anaesthesia in high risk patients
  Analgesia for instrumental delivery and suturing
  To supplement regional anaesthesia for caesarean section
Adjunct to local and regional anaesthetic techniques
  For sedation/analgesia during nerve block
  Supplemental analgesia for an inadequate block
Day case anaesthesia
  For brief diagnostic and therapeutic procedures
  To supplement local and regional techniques
Paediatric practice
  For painful procedures (e.g. removal of drains, lumbar puncture)
  Dressing changes
  Sedation for imaging
  Orally as a premedicant
Use outside the operating room
  Burn units (e.g. debridement, dressing changes)
  Accident and emergency rooms (e.g. closed reductions)
  Intensive care units (e.g. sedation, painful procedures)
  Recovery rooms (e.g. postoperative sedation and analgesia)
  Field use (e.g. trapped casualties, battlefield use)

---

nervous system activity. Ketamine may cause a further increase in the pulmonary vascular resistance, however, with the overall haemodynamic response being very variable as a result. There is still controversy regarding the use of ketamine in patients with hypovolaemic shock. Although ketamine causes a marked pressor response in normovolaemic subjects, in the presence of severe hypovolaemia blood pressure may actually decrease. It is likely that there is a diminished catecholamine response to ketamine in critically ill patients which unmasks its direct myocardial depressant and vasodilatory effects.

Ketamine has beneficial effects on airway resistance in patients with reactive airway disease and those receiving parenteral bronchodilators. It is also valuable as a maintenance agent during one-lung anaesthesia in patients with severe pulmonary disease or abnormal blood gas values. Ketamine results in improved oxygenation because of its ability to preserve the hypoxic vasoconstrictor reflex, thereby decreasing pulmonary shunt fraction. It also provides effective anaesthesia and analgesia while permitting delivery of a high inspired oxygen concentration.

In children, intramuscular ketamine (4–8 mg/kg) may be useful for induction of anaesthesia and for diagnostic and minor surgical procedures. Ketamine can also be given orally to children to produce sedation. A dose of approximately 6 mg/kg is required and produces predictable sedation within 20–25 min without significant side effects.

Ketamine isomers

Ketamine is currently available as a racemic mixture containing both S(+) and R(−) ketamine enantiomers mixed in an equal ratio. In animals, the S(+) isomer of ketamine produces more prolonged hypnosis, more profound analgesia, and less postanaesthetic excitement compared to the R(−) isomer or the racemate.[26, 27] Similar effects were observed in humans, with more effective anaesthesia, fewer psychic emergence reactions, and less agitated behaviour following S(+) ketamine compared to racemic or R(−) ketamine.[19] In addition, S(+) ketamine had a more beneficial effect on postoperative pain.[19]

The pharmacokinetic and pharmacodynamic data comparing racemic ketamine and S(+) ketamine suggest that S(+) offers better controllability because the clearance of S(+) ketamine is higher than the racemic mixture and the concentration–effect curve is steeper. This should make the titration of S(+) ketamine to clinical effects somewhat easier compared to the racemic mixture. In addition, there appears to be an interaction between the two optical isomers, with the clearance of S(+) ketamine being reduced in the presence of R(−) ketamine. This interaction may explain the more rapid recovery observed after S(+) compared to the racemate.[21] It remains to be seen whether S(+) ketamine will be made commercially available.

In summary, ketamine is a very versatile drug and remains useful in certain clinical situations. Its more widespread use is limited by delayed recovery, emergence phenomena, and a variety of stimulatory effects, which result in increases in systemic arterial, intraocular, and intracranial pressures. While benzodiazepine pretreatment can modify or even prevent some of these adverse effects, others are more resistant to modification. It has long been known that ketamine is a racemic mixture and that most of its beneficial properties are produced by the S(+) optical isomer. It is now relatively more easy to produce single optical isomers in large quantities and so greater interest has been shown in S(+) ketamine. Although this compound is potentially a more useful drug than the racemic form, it is currently unclear whether it has sufficient advantages to make its further development commercially worthwhile.

Etomidate

Etomidate is an imidazole derivative with potent and short acting hypnotic properties. Although etomidate is presented as a racemic mixture, only the (+) isomer is anaesthetically active. Etomidate is insoluble in water and was originally dissolved in cremophor EL. After the problems of that solvent became known, etomidate was reformulated in 35% propylene glycol and has been commercially available in that form since 1977. The low pH (5·6) and high osmolality (4600 mOsm/l) of propylene glycol result in a number of problems, however, including pain on injection and thrombophlebitis. This problem appears to have been solved by the suspension of etomidate in lipofundin, a lipid emulsion. This preparation of etomidate is now becoming available in several European countries. Etomidate is about six times more potent than methohexitone and approximately 25 times more potent than thiopentone. It appears to be somewhat safer than other anaesthetics, with a therapeutic index (LD_{50}/ ED_{50}) of 26 compared to 9·5 for methohexitone and 4·6 for thiopentone (in rats).

Pharmacokinetics

The major pharmacokinetic values for etomidate are shown in comparison to other iv hypnotic agents in table 3.1. Etomidate is approximately 65% bound to plasma proteins, predominantly albumin. Its volume of distribution at steady state is reported as 2·5–4·5 l/kg with an initial distribution half-life of 2·8 min, a redistribution half life of about 28 min and an elimination half life of 2·9–5·3 h.[28] Similar pharmacokinetic values have been reported for the new lipid formulation of etomidate.

Etomidate rapidly penetrates the blood–brain barrier with peak levels at the effect site occurring within one minute of administration, corresponding to the fast onset of hypnosis. Etomidate undergoes rapid ester hydrolysis in the liver to its major (carboxylic acid) metabolite, which is pharmacologically inactive. In humans, 75% of an iv dose is excreted as the metabolite in the urine during the first 24 h and about 13% is excreted in faeces.

Pharmacodynamics

The effects of etomidate on a variety of organ systems are summarised in comparison to other iv hypnotics in table 3.2.

CNS effects   The EEG effects of etomidate are similar to those produced by thiopentone and methohexitone. Etomidate's main site of action appears to lie within the neocortex and its primary effects may occur by inhibition of the GABA-adrenergic system. A high incidence of myoclonus is observed during induction of anaesthesia with etomidate in the absence of premedication. This probably occurs through disinhibition of the extrapyramidal system, which regulates involuntary movements. This myoclonic activity can be reduced somewhat by pretreatment with opioids and/or benzodiazepines. Myoclonic activity should not be confused with epileptogenic seizures. Nevertheless, as with propofol, poorly substantiated case reports have led to the suggestion that etomidate is "epileptogenic". Epileptic attacks occur far less frequently during etomidate anaesthesia than would be expected if it possessed significant convulsant activity. No clinical or EEG signs of epileptic seizures have been observed in patients without a previous history of epilepsy receiving etomidate. Even in epileptic patients, clear EEG evidence of convulsant activity has not been observed during etomidate anaesthesia. Indeed, etomidate has been shown to possess anticonvulsant properties in some experimental animals.

Etomidate can safely be used for induction of anaesthesia in patients with increased ICP. It lowers both CBF and $CMRO_2$. The latter is reduced somewhat more (45%) than the former (36%), and cerebral perfusion pressure is well maintained.[29]

CVS effects Etomidate has minimal effects on haemodynamics and myocardial function in healthy patients. The usual induction dose produces about a 10% reduction in MAP, primarily through reduced peripheral vascular resistance. Heart rate and cardiac index typically increase by 10% while stroke volume, left ventricular end diastolic pressure (LVEDP), and contractility remain relatively unchanged after an induction dose of etomidate. Even in patients with moderate cardiac dysfunction, etomidate (0·3 mg/kg) produces only minor cardiovascular changes, typically 8–10% decreases in cardiac index.

The increase in heart rate seen with etomidate produces a slight increase in myocardial oxygen consumption. This is more than compensated for by decreased coronary vascular resistance and a 20% increase in coronary perfusion, reducing arteriovenous O_2 extraction and maintaining the oxygen supply and demand ratio. The minimal negative inotropic effects of etomidate compared to alternative currently available iv induction agents make it the drug of choice in patients with preexisting cardiovascular disease.

Respiratory system effects Etomidate has minimal ventilatory depressant properties. Apnoea occurs less frequently with etomidate compared to thiopentone, methohexitone or propofol. Unusually among iv induction agents, etomidate may increase the minute ventilation.

Effects on other organ systems Etomidate has minimal effect on renal or hepatic function. Intraocular pressure is reduced by approximately 60% after an induction dose of etomidate. It has been safely used in humans during pregnancy without reports of adverse effects.

In 1983, a report was published describing substantially increased mortality in a group of ICU patients sedated with etomidate.[30] Mortality was associated with low cortisol levels and was attributed to etomidate induced suppression of adrenal cortisol synthesis. Etomidate has subsequently been shown to be a potent inhibitor of 11-β hydroxylase in the adrenal cortex,[31] even after an induction dose. This effect is relatively shortlived (6-8 h), however, and probably of little clinical significance. There is still some degree of uncertainty regarding the potential effects of etomidate on the stress response to surgery and on patient outcome. The consensus view is that it is safe when used as an induction agent and also when used for maintenance as part of a TIVA technique, even in critically ill patients. Furthermore, it should be remembered that other commonly used drugs (e.g. opioid analgesics) can also depress plasma cortisol levels.

Miscellaneous effects Pain on injection of etomidate occurs frequently. As with propofol, the incidence varies with the size and site of the veins used and can be reduced somewhat by preadministration of fentanyl or lignocaine. In addition to causing pain, etomidate can also cause thrombophlebitis, which may persist for several days. This takes the form of a hard painful vein proximal to the site of injection, appearing 3–4 days after administration. Interestingly, the occurrence of thrombophlebitis bears no relationship to the intensity of the pain on injection. These venous sequelae of etomidate are related to its formulation in propylene glycol and can be modified by the use of alternative solvents. Pain on injection is significantly reduced by the use of polyethylene glycol, although this formulation is insufficiently stable for commercial use. Pain is also reduced, but not abolished, by the use of hydroxypropyl-β-cyclodextrin.[32] Etomidate has also been prepared in lipofundin, which appears to prevent all the venous side effects. In a comparative study, 36% of the patients receiving etomidate in propylene glycol described the injection as painful.[33] Three patients had already developed a venous thrombosis by the first postoperative day, while a further nine out of the 47 patients studied had some tenderness on palpation of the vein and by the seventh day, nine patients had a thrombosis. In contrast, no patient had injection pain or any sign of venous irritation when etomidate was administered in lipofundin.[33] The use of lipofundin does not alter the bioavailability of etomidate compared to propylene glycol, and the same cardiovascular stability is maintained.[33]

Interestingly, the incidence of myoclonic activity following injection of etomidate in lipofundin has been reported as 10%. This is lower than in previous studies when etomidate was dissolved in propylene glycol and the incidence of this side effect may also have been reduced by reformulation.[34] Etomidate in lipofundin is now available for clinical use in some parts of Europe as Etomidate Lipuro™.

Nausea and vomiting are common side effects after etomidate with an incidence of 30–40%. PONV has been a major factor limiting the use of etomidate for day case surgery. This side effect may also be reduced by reformulation in lipid.

Injecting etomidate in propylene glycol results in a transient haemolysis probably due to the high osmolality of the solvent (4965 mOsm). While this is unlikely to cause detectable renal injury in healthy patients, significant haemolysis and haemoglobinuria may occur in patients with preexisting renal disease or in association with intraoperative autotransfusion and other drugs causing haemolysis. Because haemolysis is a direct consequence of the high osmolality of etomidate in propylene glycol, the lipofundin preparation of etomidate should not cause this problem as it has a near physiologic osmolality of 400 mOsm/l.

In summary, the reformulation of etomidate in lipofundin emulsion appears to retain the beneficial cardiovascular properties of etomidate while reducing or eliminating many of its unpleasant side effects. These developments make etomidate a more attractive intravenous hypnotic agent and it is likely that its use will increase in the future.

Barbiturates

Several members of the barbiturate family have previously been used as iv anaesthetics, although only thiopentone and methohexitone are still in common use. Commonly described as ultrashort acting, the hypnotic effects of these barbiturates are shortlived after a small bolus because of rapid redistribution. Thiopentone and methohexitone rapidly accumulate following repeat dosing, however, due to a relatively small central compartment and an elimination half life of several hours, limiting their usefulness.

Physicochemical properties

Thiopentone and methohexitone are derivatives of barbituric acid, which is pharmacologically inert. Substitution at positions 1 and 2 of the barbituric acid molecule results in a number of compounds with anaesthetic properties. Both thiopentone and methohexitone have hydrogen atom substitutions at position 1 of the molecule. In addition, thiopentone is a thiobarbiturate with a sulphur substitution at position 2, while methohexitone is an oxybarbiturate with an oxygen substitution at position 2.

Thiopentone was introduced as an induction agent in 1934 and is the oldest iv anaesthetic still in common use. Methohexitone was introduced in 1957. Both are useful for induction of anaesthesia because of rapid onset of action. These drugs are highly lipid soluble with slightly alkaline pKa values (7·6 for thiopentone and 7·9 for methohexitone), which permit them to rapidly cross the blood–brain barrier. Both agents are weak acids and virtually insoluble in water. Their sodium salts are water soluble, but are strongly alkaline in aqueous solutions (pH > 10). As a result, they will cause considerable tissue damage if injected subcutaneously or intraarterially and will precipitate (causing occlusion of intravenous tubing) when mixed with most other agents including suxamethonium. One advantage of the high pH is a degree of bacteriostatic activity, allowing the drugs to be kept in solution for up to two weeks.

Mechanism of action

In common with other anaesthetics, the mechanism of action of the barbiturates is not fully understood. They affect many neurotransmitter systems, although their actions at the $GABA_A$ receptor correlate with anaesthetic potency and are stereospecific. It is therefore most likely that the anaesthetic properties of these drugs are due to effects on the $GABA_A$ receptor and subsequent effects on voltage sensitive sodium channels.

Pharmacokinetics

The major pharmacokinetic values for the barbiturates are shown in comparison to other iv hypnotic agents in table 3.1. Thiopentone and methohexitone are highly protein bound to plasma albumin. As thiopentone clearance is directly related to unbound thiopentone levels, it will be affected by changes in albumin levels, as well as by drugs which displace thiopentone from albumin. However, changes in thiopentone's elimination are unlikely to be clinically relevant when it is used solely for induction of anaesthesia. The volume of distribution of the central compartment (VC) for thiopentone ranges from 8 to 26 l for adults. Thiopentone's fast onset probably occurs because the brain is part of a small volume that rapidly equilibrates with thiopentone in the central compartment blood. The effect site rate constant (k_{e0}) value for thiopentone is 0·3/min, while that for methohexitone is 0·6/min. The steady state volumes of distribution (Vd_{ss}) of thiopentone and methohexitone are 2·5 and 2·2 l/kg, respectively.

Thiopentone and methohexitone are both eliminated predominantly via the liver with very little renal involvement. The elimination clearance (Cl_e) for thiopentone is 250 ml/min, while that for methohexitone is considerably greater at 690 ml/min. The hepatic extraction of methohexitone (50–87%) is considerably greater than that of thiopentone (10–20%). As a result, methohexitone's elimination half life (3·9 h) is less than half that of thiopentone (11·6 h). The elimination of methohexitone is also more dependent on hepatic blood flow (and therefore more variable) compared to thiopentone. Nevertheless, the shortlived clinical effects of methohexitone are still predominantly due to redistribution, just as with thiopentone. At high blood concentrations, the elimination of thiopentone becomes zero order, dependent on the capacity of the hepatic P_{450} system.

For this reason, thiopentone is not a good choice of iv anaesthetic for prolonged infusion. After a two hour infusion designed to produce constant plasma concentrations of thiopentone, the time required for a 25% decrease in concentration is only slightly over 15 min. In contrast, the time required for a 50% drop (context sensitive half time) exceeds one hour, while the time for a 75% fall in the blood concentration is more than two hours. As a result of its more rapid hepatic elimination, the context sensitive half time of methohexitone is 20 min or less for infusion durations likely to be used in clinical anaesthesia. Methohexitone is therefore more appro-

47

priate for infusion than thiopentone, but has also been largely displaced by propofol.

Pharmacodynamics

The effects of the barbiturates on a variety of organ systems are summarised in comparison to other iv hypnotics in table 3.2.

CNS effects The barbiturates cause depression of cerebral electrical activity and cerebral metabolism. Thiopentone depresses $CMRO_2$ in a dose dependent manner to a maximum of 55% of conscious levels. The reduced $CMRO_2$ causes cerebral vasoconstriction, reducing CBF and ICP. Because ICP is reduced more than MAP, however, CPP remains normal or is slightly elevated. Thiopentone reduces neuronal activity, resulting in a dose dependent depression of the EEG. The EEG amplitude increases and frequency decreases, producing a burst suppression pattern, changing to isoelectricity at the point of maximally depressed $CMRO_2$. Thiopentone is an effective anticonvulsant, whereas methohexitone has proconvulsant properties and may cause seizures in undiagnosed epileptics.

CVS effects Thiopentone predominantly produces venodilation, causing blood to pool in the periphery. Systemic vascular resistance and arterial blood pressure usually remain relatively unaltered following normal induction doses in healthy patients. At high doses, thiopentone directly depresses myocardial contractility. Both thiopentone and methohexitone increase heart rate via the baroreceptor reflex, the increase with methohexitone (40%) being greater than with thiopentone (25%). As with other iv induction agents, great care is required in patients with hypovolaemic shock and heart failure in whom cardiovascular function may be maintained by considerably increased sympathetic tone. Greater haemodynamic changes (e.g. decreased afterload, left ventricular stroke work index, coronary blood flow, myocardial oxygen consumption) can also be expected in patients with ischaemic heart disease.

Respiratory system effects Both thiopentone and methohexitone are dose dependent ventilatory depressants, and apnoea usually follows an induction dose in most patients. The responses to hypoxaemia and hypercapnia are also depressed, as are protective airway reflexes, although not to a degree sufficient to permit tracheal intubation or insertion of a laryngeal mask airway (LMA), as is observed with propofol.

Renal and hepatic system effects Normal anaesthetic induction doses cause no significant changes in liver function, even in the presence of preexisting liver disease. Thiopentone may decrease renal blood flow and urine output although clinically significant decreases are unlikely with correct fluid management. Patients who are cirrhotic, uraemic or on chronic dialysis will have reduced protein binding of thiopentone. The induction dose should be administered more slowly to prevent excessively high "free" thiopentone levels. As a greater proportion of free drug is available to the liver for metabolism, the clinical duration of thiopentone may be reduced, provided that liver function is normal.

Miscellaneous effects Thiobarbiturates (but not oxybarbiturates) cause dose dependent histamine release. Clinically significant haemodynamic or pulmonary changes are rarely observed, although thiopentone occasionally causes anaphylaxis. Thiopentone decreases plasma cortisol concentrations, but does not prevent the stress response to surgery. Pain on injection is common with methohexitone but it is rare with thiopentone unless extravasation occurs. Subcutaneous or intraarterial injection of thiopentone causes pain, oedema, erythema, and reactions ranging from discomfort to tissue necrosis and gangrene, especially with more concentrated solutions. Misplacement of methohexitone is much less harmful.

Involuntary muscular movements, coughing or hiccuping occur commonly following induction of anaesthesia with methohexitone but are less common after thiopentone. Barbiturates can precipitate attacks of acute intermittent or variegate porphyria in susceptible patients by inducing the production of δ-aminolevulinic acid synthetase, the catalyst to the rate limiting step in porphyrin synthesis. Barbiturate administration induces a number of symptoms of nervous system dysfunction, including paralysis, abdominal pain, and photosensitivity.

In summary, thiopentone is still used as an induction agent in situations where rapid recovery is not important. Methohexitone is commonly used as a single bolus dose for ECT because of its well established effects on the convulsive response. Neither barbiturate is now commonly used as a maintenance agent because of prolonged recovery, especially following thiopentone.

Benzodiazepines

The benzodiazepines produce a broad spectrum of CNS effects including hypnosis, anxiolysis, and amnesia. Although they have multiple clinical uses, in anaesthesia they are employed predominantly for premedication, to reduce the possibility of intraoperative awareness, and for conscious sedation. The benzodiazepines act by occupying the GABA benzodiazepine receptor, facilitating the inhibitory action of gamma-amino butyric acid (GABA) on neuronal transmission. This interaction accounts for the anxiolytic, anticonvulsant, and muscle relaxation effects of benzodiazepines, but the hypnotic effects are probably mediated elsewhere.

Both diazepam and lorazepam have been used as premedicant drugs for the relief of anxiety. Both are long lasting, however, with the potential to delay recovery. Diazepam has also been used as an iv induction agent, although slow onset, delayed recovery, and a high incidence of venous thrombosis have limited its use. An important development, therefore, was the synthesis of midazolam, a water soluble, short acting benzodiazepine, 2–3 times more potent than diazepam.

Pharmacokinetics

The major pharmacokinetic values for midazolam are shown in comparison to other iv hypnotic agents in table 3.1. Midazolam is water soluble with a pKa of 6·15 and is extensively (96%) bound to albumin. It has a distribution half life of 5–10 min and an elimination half life of 2–4 h. Midazolam has a clearance of 6–10 ml/kg/min, greater than diazepam and lorazepam. Consequently, midazolam has a relatively short duration of clinical effect when delivered by bolus or short infusion, although it becomes longer acting following more prolonged administration. There are no significant active metabolites of midazolam, in contrast to other benzodiazepines. Approximately 50% of an orally administered dose of midazolam reaches the circulation and this drug is increasingly being used as an oral premedicant, despite the lack of a commercial oral preparation.

Pharmacodynamics

The effects of midazolam on a variety of organ systems are summarised in comparison to other iv hypnotics in table 3.2.

CNS effects Midazolam causes a dose related reduction in cerebral metabolism and blood flow and has been used as an induction agent in patients with decreased intracranial compliance. Induction is relatively slow, however, with the risk of hypoxia and hypercarbia during the gradual loss of consciousness. Midazolam, in common with other benzodiazepines, raises the seizure threshold somewhat.

CVS effects When used for induction of anaesthesia, midazolam causes a relatively mild and transient hypotensive effect, although this is more marked compared to diazepam. Nevertheless, midazolam (0·2 mg/kg) has been used safely in patients with severe aortic stenosis. The hypotensive effects of midazolam are greater in the presence of severe hypovolaemia and may also be exaggerated when coadministered with opioids, due to a reduction in resting sympathetic tone and decreased catecholamine release.

Respiratory system effects Midazolam causes a relatively minor depression of central respiratory drive. Respiratory depression is more profound in patients with chronic obstructive pulmonary disease, and midazolam (and other benzodiazepines) has a synergistic respiratory depressant effect when given with opioids (see chapter 5).

Clinical applications

Clinically, midazolam is often used as a preanaesthetic medication. It acts rapidly following iv administration (2–3 min) and produces profound amnesia lasting 20–30 min. Intravenous midazolam can significantly reduce the dose of other iv drugs required to induce anaesthesia and the concept of coinduction has gained in popularity recently. For premedication before iv access is established, midazolam may be given intramuscularly or orally. Currently, oral administration requires the use of the iv solution, usually mixed with fruit syrup (ibuprofen syrup provides both flavour and prophylactic analgesia) to mask its bitter taste. There is no commercially available oral midazolam preparation at present.

Midazolam can also be used for iv induction of anaesthesia, requiring a dose of 0·2–0·3 mg/kg in unpremedicated patients. When delivered over 30–60 s, loss of consciousness occurs in less than two minutes, although this is slower than other iv induction drugs. Following repeat doses or prolonged infusions, midazolam may accumulate, leading to delayed recovery. This may be problematic when midazolam is used as a maintenance anaesthetic or for conscious sedation and especially when it is used to provide sedation on the ICU.

Steroid anaesthetics

A number of naturally occurring steroids belonging to the pregnane and androstane groups have been shown to have anaesthetic properties. There appears to be no relationship between hypnotic (anaesthetic) and hormonal properties, however. Indeed, the most potent anaesthetic steroid, pregnane-3,20-dione (pregnanedione), is virtually devoid of endocrine activity.

As many of the naturally occurring (and most of the early synthetic) anaesthetic steroids were water insoluble, practical application awaited the synthesis of water soluble steroids. Hydroxydione was the first potentially useful anaesthetic steroid. It was derived from pregnanedione and made water soluble by esterification at the C21 position. In clinical practice, hydroxydione produced slow but smooth induction of anaesthesia, accompanied by minimal changes in cardiorespiratory function, good muscle relaxation, and a pleasant recovery.[35] Unfortunately, it was associated with a high incidence of pain on injection as well as quite severe thrombophlebitis, which led to its abandonment. Nevertheless, the experience with hydroxydione increased enthusiasm in the search for better anaesthetic steroids. A number of promising compounds were synthesised, which had rapid onset of action and the high therapeutic indices characteristic of all steroid anaesthetics. Side effects such as paraesthesia and convulsant properties were problematic, however.

Following hydroxydione, the next most important steroid anaesthetic was Althesin. This was a mixture of two steroids, alphaxalone and alphadolone, both of which had anaesthetic activity but were virtually insoluble in water. Alphaxalone was the more potent of the two steroids, and alphadolone was primarily present to increase the solubility of alphaxalone in cremophor EL. Like other steroids, Althesin is thought to have exerted its anaesthetic effects by way of interaction with the GABA$_A$ receptor–chloride channel complex. Benzodiazepines and barbiturates have also been shown to have effects on these structures. Clinically, Althesin had a rapid onset and short duration of effect. It had a high therapeutic index with minimal CVS depression, even at twice the ED$_{50}$ induction dose. It caused a brief period of hyperventilation following induction of anaesthesia and also caused a beneficial reduction in ICP. Althesin had a number of other advantages, including minimal effects on renal and hepatic function, safety in patients susceptible to malignant hyperpyrexia (but not porphyria), decrease in intraocular pressure, and a relaxant effect on laryngeal muscle. Its major advantage, however, was a more rapid recovery compared to the barbiturates.

Regrettably, Althesin resulted in a number of adverse reactions including peripheral vasodilation, skin flushes, oedema, and wheals from a histaminoid reaction. Repeat exposure to Althesin occasionally resulted in more severe cardiovascular collapse, mediated via classic complement pathway activation. The detection of IgG antibodies to cremophor EL suggests that the solvent was responsible and not the individual steroids.[36] The incidence of adverse reactions to Althesin ranged from 1 in 1000 to 1 in 18 000, but could be as high as 1 in 14 following a previous exposure. As a result of these adverse events, Althesin was never marketed in the United States and was withdrawn from clinical use in the United Kingdom in 1984. To date, attempts to find an acceptable alternative solvent for alphaxalone have been unsuccessful.

Recent developments in steroid anaesthesia

Both progesterone and 5α-pregnanedione have hypnotic activity. It has been shown that both of these compounds are metabolised to 3α-OH, 5α-pregnan-20-one (pregnanolone), and it is this metabolite which is anaesthetically active. Subsequently, pregnanolone in a lipid emulsion (eltanolone) has been intensively investigated as an iv anaesthetic. Pregnanolone emulsion induces anaesthesia with minimal haemodynamic effects and only mild ventilatory depression. Compared with propofol, eltanolone causes less pain on injection.[37] Recovery from eltanolone was somewhat slower than that following propofol,[38] suggesting that the clinical place of eltanolone was not likely to be as an alternative iv anaesthetic for brief day case procedures. The lack of a clear clinical advantage of eltanolone, combined with a relatively high incidence of allergic type reactions (e.g. rashes, urticaria), resulted in the withdrawal of eltanolone from further clinical development in 1996.

A number of water soluble steroid anaesthetics have also been investigated. Minaxolone, studied during the 1970s, had some properties similar to Althesin, although induction and recovery were somewhat slower. It was withdrawn following a high incidence of excitatory side effects during induction. Another steroid, ORG 20599, has been found to have a therapeutic index of 13 and to be capable of inducing a short lasting hypnotic effect. The relative instability of this drug in aqueous solution has prevented evaluation in humans to date. More recently, ORG 21465, another water soluble 2-substituted aminosteroid, has been evaluated in animals and humans. This steroid also has a high therapeutic index but is once more associated with a high incidence of excitatory effects. Its future is currently unclear. Indeed, despite the potential for an anaesthetic with a high therapeutic index and smooth, brief duration anaesthesia, the future of steroid anaesthesia is currently rather bleak.

Opioid and non-opioid analgesics

Opioid analgesics

The opioids are by far the oldest known group of drugs still used in modern anaesthesia. Opium was first described in the third century BC. It is derived from the oriental poppy (*Papaver somniferum*) and contains more than 20 different alkaloids, of which morphine is the major component. A number of opium alkaloids have been isolated, including morphine (from Morpheus, the Greek god of dreams), codeine, and papaverine. These opium derivatives are referred to as *opiates*, while the term *opioid* is used to refer to synthetic drugs with morphine-like properties. The term *narcotic* is sometimes still used interchangeably with opioids, although it non-specifically describes sedation and sleep resulting from any drug, being derived from the Greek word for stupor.

The use of opioids to provide perioperative analgesia predates the development of general anaesthesia. After the introduction of the first volatile anaesthetics, morphine was used as a premedicant and was found to decrease chloroform requirements. Subsequent attempts were made to use large doses of morphine with scopolamine to provide anaesthesia as an alternative to inhaled agents. While this reduced excitation during induction and emergence, patient movement and severe ventilatory depression proved problematic.[39] As a consequence, the early opioids were used mainly as adjuvants to inhalational agents or regional anaesthetic techniques.

The first synthetic opioid to be produced was pethidine (meperidine), which appeared in 1938. By 1947 it was being used as part of a balanced technique along with N_2O, curare, and barbiturates. Both morphine and pethidine were used in high doses with oxygen for cardiac anaesthesia.

53

Although a degree of haemodynamic stability was achieved in patients with compromised cardiovascular function, it was not always possible to prevent intraoperative hypertension, and intraoperative recall was common with both drugs. In addition, morphine was also associated with histamine related hypotension, while tachycardia and cardiac depression complicated the use of pethidine.

In 1953, Paul Janssen began to search for more potent opioids in the belief that greater potency would enhance specificity, reduce side effects, and improve safety. This research led to the synthesis of fentanyl (in 1960), which was 100–300 times as potent as morphine, with a higher therapeutic index and fewer side effects. Fentanyl found early use in combination with droperidol in neurolept analgesia and with N_2O in neurolept anaesthesia (chapter 2). Fentanyl was also widely used in cardiac anaesthesia. It was more effective as a sole anaesthetic agent than either morphine or pethidine, although it too resulted in intraoperative awareness and delayed recovery when used alone and is now more commonly used as part of a balanced technique. Further developments produced sufentanil (mid 1970s) which is ten times as potent as fentanyl and has a shorter duration of action. Alfentanil was introduced in the late 1970s. It is five times less potent than fentanyl, but of faster onset and much shorter duration. The latest development is remifentanil, which is approximately equipotent to fentanyl. It is unique in having an ester structure which is rapidly metabolised by blood and tissue non-specific esterases, resulting in an ultrashort duration of action.

The opioids exert their effects by interaction with stereoselective transmembrane opioid receptors which exist to bind endogenous opioid peptides. Three receptor subtypes have been identified, termed μ, κ and δ. In addition, ε and σ receptors also bind opioids, although they bind non-opioid drugs (e.g. ketamine) as well. The majority of the clinical effects (beneficial and otherwise) of morphine-like compounds are mediated via μ receptors. Two subpopulations are recognised: μ-1 mediates analgesia while μ-2 mediates ventilatory depression.[40] This raises the possibility (as yet unrealised) of developing specific μ-1 receptor agonists capable of producing analgesia without ventilatory depression. κ receptors are concentrated in those areas of the spinal cord and brain which modulate afferent nociceptive impulses. A pure κ-agonist might be useful clinically as these drugs do not cause respiratory depression and mediate dysphoria rather than euphoria which might reduce their abuse potential. κ agonists would also produce sedation and inhibit antidiuretic hormone (ADH) release, however. The partial opioid agonists (e.g. nalorphine, pentazocine, butorphanol, nalbuphine, dezocine) probably provide analgesia via κ receptors. These drugs are also probably partial agonists at the μ receptor, however, and are therefore still able to produce ventilatory depression. δ receptors are located spinally and supraspinally, where they bind enkepha-

Table 3.4   Major pharmacokinetic parameters for the opioid analgesics and opioid antagonists

Drug	Protein binding (%)	V_C (l/kg)	Vd_{ss} (l/kg)	Clearance (ml/kg/min)
Morphine	23–26	-	3–5	15–20
Pethidine	70	1–2	3–5	8–18
Codeine	7–25	-	2·5–3·5	10–15
Fentanyl	80	0·5–1·0	3–5	10–20
Sufentanil	93	0·2	2·5–3·0	10–15
Alfentanil	90	0·1–0·3	0·4–1·0	4–9
Remifentanil	70	0·1–0·2	0·3–0·4	40–60
Naloxone	40	-	2·6–3	20–30
Naltrexone	20	-	16	20
Nalmephene	-	-	2·3	14

V_C Volume of central compartment; Vd_{ss} Volume of distribution at steady state

lins. Activation of these receptors may enhance analgesia by modulating μ receptor activity.

Pharmacokinetics

The main pharmacokinetic parameters of the opioid analgesics are summarised in table 3.4. Oral absorption of morphine-like compounds is slow with a high degree of first pass metabolism. Morphine has a bioavailability of only 20%, although that of codeine is somewhat higher at 60%. Following intramuscular (im) administration, peak plasma concentrations of morphine occur 7–20 min after injection, while pethidine takes about 30 min to reach its peak effect. There is also a large interpatient variability in peak concentration after im absorption. Morphine is relatively little bound to plasma proteins (approximately 25%). Following iv administration, the plasma concentration rapidly declines, described by a bi- or triexponential decay function. Because morphine is relatively hydrophilic, it traverses the blood–brain barrier relatively slowly and concentrations of morphine in the CNS lag significantly behind serum concentrations. In fact, peak CSF concentration may not occur until 15–30 min after intravenous administration, which makes it difficult to titrate the optimal dose of morphine in order to achieve adequate analgesia without sedative or respiratory depressant effects. Morphine is also slow to leave the CSF because of the increased ionised fraction of morphine in the relatively acidic CSF. The clinical effects of morphine are therefore longer lasting than would be expected from its plasma pharmacokinetics. These discrepancies between serum levels and clinical effects are far greater for morphine than for the other, more lipophilic opioids. Morphine is primarily cleared by hepatic metabolism, with typical clearance of 15–23 ml/kg/min. Morphine is metabolised very rapidly to morphine-3-glucuronide and morphine-6-glucuronide. The latter metabolite is highly active and is eliminated more slowly from the CSF than the parent compound. With prolonged morphine administration, morphine-6-glucuronide probably contributes significantly to both analgesia and ventilatory depression.

Sufentanil, fentanyl, alfentanil, and remifentanil are all more potent than morphine. They also differ in their time to peak effect and in their clinical duration of action so that varying dosage schedules are required, as well as different relative doses, when changing from one opioid to another. Approximately 80% of fentanyl is bound to plasma proteins, and it has a high lipid solubility. This results in a large volume of distribution (3–6 l/kg). Fentanyl equilibrates much more rapidly with the CSF following iv administration compared to morphine, although brain levels still lag approximately five minutes behind the plasma concentration. Fentanyl's high lipid solubility and volume of distribution contribute to considerable interpatient variability in peak plasma levels after intravenous administration, as well as other pharmacokinetic parameters. Fentanyl also has a high clearance (10–20 ml/kg/min). Fentanyl is primarily metabolised in the liver (by N-dealkylation and hydroxylation) to norfentanyl and other relatively inactive metabolites.

Sufentanil is approximately ten times as potent as fentanyl, approximately twice as lipid soluble and highly bound (93%) to plasma proteins. Sufentanil's pharmacokinetics conform to a three compartment model, with an apparent volume of distribution at steady state of approximately 3 l/kg and hepatic clearance of 3 ml/kg/min. Sufentanil is metabolised by a variety of hepatic pathways to inactive metabolites. It has a shorter duration of effect compared to fentanyl and is comparable to alfentanil provided that the duration of infusion is less than 6–8 h. This is probably the result of a high degree of plasma protein binding and lower volume of distribution.

Alfentanil is also highly protein bound (90%), like other synthetic opioids, mostly to $\alpha 1$ acid glycoproteins. Alfentanil enters the CNS effect site more rapidly than fentanyl, despite lower lipid solubility. This low lipid affinity prevents much uptake of alfentanil by non-specific CNS tissue, however, resulting in a shorter duration of clinical effect. Although the clearance of alfentanil (4–9 ml/min/kg) is less than that of fentanyl, this is offset by a smaller volume of distribution (0·4–1·0 l/kg), limiting distribution and tissue accumulation. Alfentanil is metabolised via similar pathways to sufentanil, producing several inactive metabolites.

Remifentanil is a new, potent synthetic opioid with a rapid onset of effect. It is unique in that it contains an ester linkage which undergoes rapid and widespread extrahepatic hydrolysis by non-specific blood and tissue esterases. Deesterification produces a carboxylic acid metabolite (GI90291) which is 300–1000 times less potent than the parent compound. The volume of distribution of remifentanil at steady state (22 l) is similar to that of alfentanil (38 l). Remifentanil's pattern of decay can be described by a three compartment model with a strikingly high clearance (4·1–5·0 l/min) which is far more important in terminating its clinical effect than its redistribution. Remifentanil's major metabolite is not subject to extra-hepatic hydrolysis and therefore has a much lower clearance. At steady state, the concentration of the metabolite is thought to be 12 times greater than that of remifentanil.[41] This should be of little significance as the metabolite is at least 300 times less potent than the parent compound. The possibility of significant metabolite accumulation in patients with renal failure is yet to be fully excluded, however. The most exciting aspect of the clearance of remifentanil is that the ester hydrolysis appears totally independent of dose, age, administration duration, renal and hepatic function, and even genetic variability. Upon stopping a remifentanil infusion, the plasma concentration decreases by a half in only three minutes, irrespective of whether the drug has been infused for minutes or hours. Clinical recovery from remifentanil infusions has been shown to be relatively independent of the administered dose. Times to awakening and spontaneous ventilation were almost identical following three hours of remifentanil-N_2O anaesthesia, despite an 80-fold difference between the highest and lowest infusion rates studied.[42]

The complex interaction of volume of distribution, clearance, and elimination all impact on the rate of recovery from opioid effects when infusions of varying duration are terminated. These effects are best described by the context sensitive half time (fig 1.3). For all the opioids, duration of administration has a major effect on rate of recovery with the single exception of remifentanil, which is shortlived under all circumstances examined to date.

Hepatic disease alters the sensitivity to opioid analgesics, a well as their distribution and elimination. With moderately impaired hepatic function, there is usually little need to reduce initial doses of opioids unless encephalopathy is present. In contrast, patients known to have very heavy alcohol consumption may require increased doses. Liver disease may result in prolonged duration of opioid action, however, and maintenance doses should be decreased accordingly. Because of its unique form of metabolism, remifentanil may be relatively immune to these problems and is likely to become the opioid of choice in severe hepatic disease.

Renal disease will result in the accumulation of opioid metabolites in proportion to the degree of renal impairment. For opioids with active metabolites (e.g. morphine, pethidine), this may result in prolonged effects and/or increased toxicity. Fentanyl and sufentanil pharmacokinetics are relatively unaffected by renal disease, although greater interpatient variability than usual may be observed. An increase in clinical effect of alfentanil may occur due to a decreased volume of distribution and an increase in the free drug fraction.[43] As the clearance of alfentanil is unlikely to be altered by renal impairment, no delay should be expected in recovery. Remifentanil's pharmacokinetics are little altered by renal insufficiency, with similar clearances in renal dialysis patients (36 ml/kg/min) and healthy volunteers

(34 ml/kg/min).[44] The remifentanil metabolite may accumulate in renal failure, but has not yet been shown to produce any significant activity or toxicity under these circumstances.

Pharmacodynamics

The opioids have wide ranging effects, beneficial and otherwise. They are usually administered to relieve pain, to minimise "stress" responses to noxious stimuli, and to maintain cardiovascular stability. Their use will also reduce the requirements for other anaesthetics (i.e. they have an MAC-reducing effect).

CNS effects Opioids produce dose related sedation, anxiolysis, cough suppression, and unconsciousness. Although they seem to be able to produce anaesthesia, this appears to be less reliably achieved than with other hypnotic agents and is associated with a significant incidence of perioperative awareness and recall (see chapter 4). The EEG shows high voltage slow (δ) waves (which appear to correlate with general anaesthesia) at high doses, although few effects are observed at lower doses. The opioids appear to have minimal effects on $CMRO_2$ and CBF. There is some evidence that ICP may be increased by large doses of opioids in victims of head trauma. This effect seems less likely at low doses, although any direct effect must be separated from the hypercarbia which will result if opioid induced ventilatory depression is not prevented.

CVS effects The naturally occurring opioids are associated with significant histamine release, resulting in vasodilation and hypotension. In contrast, the synthetic agents are associated with extremely stable haemodynamics, better than can be achieved by any other agents. Opioid receptors are found throughout the central and peripheral cardiovascular and sympathetic nervous system regulatory centres. The only significant cardiovascular effect of the synthetic opioids is to produce a significant slowing of the heart rate. This phenomenon is not usually associated with a significant reduction in CVS stability, however. As with other "anaesthetics", hypotension may occur during induction of anaesthesia in hypotensive, vasoconstricted individuals, while hypertension may occur in the presence of inadequate anaesthesia/analgesia.

Respiratory system effects The opioids are potent depressors of respiratory drive, as well as upper airway and tracheal reflexes. This may be beneficial during anaesthesia (and on the ICU) in helping patients to tolerate endotracheal tubes (ETTs) without coughing or "bucking". ETTs are highly stimulating and may produce hypertension, increased intracranial pressure secondary to coughing, and impaired gas exchange. The use of opioid analgesics can reduce coughing and bucking during emergence from general anaesthesia without delaying the return to consciousness.[45] The potent depression of ventilatory drive by opioids may be problematic, however. Direct depression of the medullary respiratory centre reduces its responsiveness to CO_2, increases the resting arterial PCO_2 and raises the apnoeic threshold. There is a shift towards irregular and periodic breathing, progressing to apnoea. Apnoea may occur well before unconsciousness and patients may breathe if requested to do so. These opioid effects are exacerbated in the absence of pain or other significant stimuli, as well as during normal sleep or in the presence of other anaesthetics or sedatives (e.g. midazolam). This may cause problems at the end of an opioid based anaesthetic or when opioids are used for postoperative pain relief. In contrast, inadequately treated pain can also result in hypoventilation, and a balance has to be attained between adequate analgesia and avoidance of opioid related side effects. Careful titration of dose to effect with the minimally effective analgesic dose being used is important for safety.

Opioids may reduce bronchial smooth muscle tone and may be useful in asthmatics or patients with reactive airways. They also have minimal effects on hypoxic pulmonary vasoconstriction and may be useful during one-lung anaesthesia.[46]

Miscellaneous effects Muscle rigidity commonly occurs with the potent, rapidly acting opioids. The effect appears to be dose related, occurring commonly with large doses (e.g. sufentanil 0.3 μg/kg, fentanyl 3 μg/kg, alfentanil 30 μg/kg) or with rapid bolus administration. This effect may be unpleasant for patients and may interfere with bag and mask ventilation. Other than using smaller doses of opioids, the only effective management is the concomitant use of muscle relaxants which totally abolish the muscle rigidity.

Postoperative nausea and vomiting are the most significant gastro-intestinal effects of the opioids, occurring in 15–60% of patients receiving an opioid containing balanced anaesthetic. The effect appears to be equally prevalent after all the available opioids. PONV appears problematic after opioid analgesics, although pain is also a potent cause of this side effect. The use of prophylactic antiemetics or alternative analgesic strategies to reduce opioid doses may be beneficial. As well as having a direct effect on the chemoreceptor trigger zone, the opioids also increase gastric secretions, decrease gastrointestinal activity, delay gastric emptying, and reduce lower oesophageal sphincter tone. These factors may all contribute to PONV. Opioids prolong postoperative ileus and may also increase constipation. All opioids increase biliary duct pressure by increasing tone in the sphincter of Oddi. This can produce biliary spasm and contributes to PONV.

Opioids consistently decrease the stress hormone response, although the clinical significance of this is not fully clear (see chapter 4). Pruritus is common following opioid administration, especially with prolonged use, although this can be reduced with antihistamines. Opioids have minimal effects on renal or hepatic function, although urinary retention can occur. This is more common after spinal or epidural administration, however.

Non-steroidal antiinflammatory drugs (NSAIDs)

Like the opioids, non-steroidal antiinflammatory drugs (NSAIDs) have been known for a long time. In 1829, salicin was identified as the active ingredient of willow bark and synthetic acetylsalicylic acid (aspirin) was produced by Bayer in 1899. In more recent years, a wide range of oral and injectable preparations of NSAIDs have been developed. With the advent of day case surgery there has been increased interest in the perioperative use of these drugs as they can avoid many of the unwanted side effects associated with the opioid analgesics (e.g. respiratory depression, nausea, vomiting, urinary retention, tolerance, addiction, and potential for abuse). The maximum efficacy of NSAIDs is not as great as that of the opioid analgesics, however, and these drugs also introduce their own side effects (e.g. gastrointestinal bleeding, bronchospasm, renal failure). Nevertheless, the NSAIDs may be very useful for treating pain of moderate severity and also have an important role in balanced analgesia.

Mechanisms of action

NSAIDs have long been thought to act by inhibiting the synthesis of prostaglandin in the periphery, which occurs in response to trauma and results in inflammation and sensitisation of nociceptors, causing a decreased pain threshold. It is this inhibition of prostaglandin synthesis which is also responsible for most of the side effects of the NSAIDs. There is also recent evidence to suggest that the NSAIDs have a centrally mediated role in pain modulation and some of these drugs are effective when given intrathecally. The rate of entry of parenterally administered NSAIDs into the CNS is slow, however, suggesting that their centrally mediated activity may be relatively unimportant in clinical use.

Pharmacokinetics

A number of NSAIDs can be orally administered (e.g. ibuprofen, naproxen, diclofenac). When given orally as a premedication, these drugs result in effective and long lasting postoperative analgesia. The use of well established drugs (e.g. ibuprofen) appears to result in fewer adverse effects than some of the newer, parenteral compounds (e.g. ketorolac) while still providing adequate analgesia. In the context of iv anaesthesia, however, only the parenteral NSAIDs will be considered further.

Ketorolac Ketorolac tromethamine (Toradol™) was the first parenteral NSAID licensed for postoperative analgesia when it was marketed in 1990. At 800 times the potency of aspirin, ketorolac is also the most potent NSAID currently available. Ketorolac is rapidly absorbed and undergoes negligible levels of first pass metabolism and may also be administered orally or intramuscularly, following which it takes 30–45 min to achieve maximum plasma concentrations, compared to a time to peak effect of approximately 20 min after iv administration. In common with other NSAIDs, ketorolac is extensively bound to protein (99%) and has a small volume of distribution. It competes for binding with drugs such as anticoagulants, digoxin, and methotrexate and displacement of these compounds from plasma proteins can enhance their toxic effects significantly. Plasma clearance of ketorolac ranges from 0·02 to 0·04 l/kg/h, with the majority of the drug excreted via the kidney (60% unchanged, 40% conjugated and hydroxylated, probably within the kidney rather than the liver). Ketorolac's elimination half life is 5·4 h, but clearance is reduced in the elderly and in the presence of renal dysfunction. Ketorolac both crosses the placenta and is excreted in breast milk, but in either case the levels achieved are exceedingly low compared to those of the mother.

Diclofenac Diclofenac sodium (Voltarol™) is a phenylacetic acid 100 times the potency of aspirin. It is poorly water soluble and is therefore dissolved in propylene glycol. When given intramuscularly, diclofenac has been associated with the production of sterile abscesses, while iv injection (in undiluted form) produces venous thrombosis in 60–80% of patients. Diclofenac now has a licence for intravenous administration, provided that it is diluted in at least 100 ml of intravenous fluid and infused over 30 min. Although this prevents venous sequelae, it is not a really practical form of administration and drugs like ketorolac are likely to be used more frequently when iv delivery is required. Diclofenac can also be given orally, although approximately 40% undergoes first pass metabolism. Rectal administration avoids this particular problem and results in effective and prolonged analgesia. Rectal diclofenac is commonly used in Europe, although issues relating to patient consent to this route of administration have reduced its use in recent times.

Like ketorolac, diclofenac is extensively bound to plasma proteins (99·5%) and has a low volume of distribution (0·12 l/kg). It is also predominantly excreted via the kidney, although almost entirely in conjugated forms.

Other parenterally available NSAIDs include ketoprofen (Orudis™, Oruvail™) and tenoxicam (Mobiflex™). A potential advantage of tenoxicam is its relatively slow clearance and potentially long duration of action. There are relatively few clinical trials comparing the effectiveness and duration of analgesia (as well as side effects) of these various NSAIDs when used in the perioperative period, however.

Pharmacodynamics

In contrast to the opioid analgesics, the perioperative use of NSAIDs does not appear to produce any reduction in the minimum alveolar

61

concentration (MAC) of volatile anaesthetics.[47] When used as the sole intraoperative analgesic, NSAIDs have been associated with an unacceptably high incidence of purposeful movement in response to surgical stimuli.[48] However, they may have fewer adverse cardiorespiratory effects and may provide longer lasting postoperative analgesia compared to the opioids. In addition, they may allow a more rapid recovery with less nausea and vomiting after day case surgery. The optimal use of NSAIDs may be in combination with low doses of opioids and local anaesthetics to significantly improve postoperative analgesia with fewer opioid related adverse effects. Where postoperative pain is mild to moderate, however, NSAIDs alone ($\pm$ local anaesthetics) may be sufficient, allowing opioid side effects to be prevented altogether. In reducing opioid dosage (or replacing opioids altogether) it is important that the NSAIDs do not add serious adverse effects of their own.

Adverse effects NSAIDs can have serious adverse effects on the renal, gastrointestinal, and coagulation systems when used in the perioperative period. Although anecdotal reports of death from acute renal toxicity or bleeding have appeared in the medical literature, the incidence of these events appears to be very low. Although potent drugs are usually associated with fewer adverse events than less potent ones (because less drug is needed for a given effect), this relationship does not appear to be true for the NSAIDs, probably because inhibition of prostaglandin synthesis mediates both beneficial and adverse effects.

While all NSAIDs can adversely affect renal function, most reports of perioperative renal impairment have involved patients with preexisting renal dysfunction or other risk factors for acute renal failure (e.g. hypovolaemia, sepsis, cardiac failure, cirrhosis). The concurrent use of NSAIDs with other nephrotoxic drugs (e.g. antibiotics) is also more likely to result in problems. Prostaglandins have relatively little effect on renal blood flow in the presence of adequate hydration; they become more important during hypovolaemic conditions or in the presence of cardiac failure. Adverse renal effects are also more likely with prolonged (rather than acute) administration.[49]

NSAIDs can also inhibit platelet function through inhibition of cyclo-oxygenase activity. The severity of this effect appears to vary between different NSAIDs.[50] Anecdotal reports of clinically significant perioperative bleeding have been relatively more common with ketorolac and indomethacin and relatively rare with ibuprofen. These adverse effects usually complicate the chronic administration of large doses of NSAIDs in the therapy of arthritic diseases and clinically significant gastrointestinal disturbances are rare following acute perioperative use, even when administered to fasting patients.

NSAIDs are also able to increase bronchospasm in asthmatic patients and have often been considered as contraindicated in these patients. In practice, only a small proportion of asthmatics suffer a worsening of their condition with NSAIDs. Because these drugs are so widely available, most asthmatics will have previously been exposed to NSAIDs and their effects will be known. In the absence of previous problems, perioperative use of NSAIDs in asthmatics appears safe. Greater caution may be required in severe asthma, however, especially when past response to NSAIDs is unknown.

In summary, there is extensive experience in the use of NSAID compounds during the perioperative period. NSAIDs have proven to be beneficial in day case surgery, as well as to supplement the opioids following major surgery. Improved pain relief and reduced opioid use have been demonstrated. Although there are clear advantages to avoiding opioids (especially in day cases), benefits from reduced opioid use have been less readily demonstrated. For example, reducing the opioid dose rarely reduces the incidence of emetic sequelae.

Although the potency of NSAIDs varies considerably, few comparative studies of their efficacy at equipotent doses have been performed. Clinical impressions suggest that the more potent drugs like ketorolac may not provide more effective analgesia, although they may have a higher incidence of adverse effects. Clearly, more work on the risks and benefits of the various NSAIDs used in the perioperative period is needed. Until then, the more established drugs like ibuprofen and diclofenac, which can be given orally or rectally, appear effective and relatively safe and should probably be used in preference to newer, systemic drugs.

Local anaesthetics

Local anaesthetics can temporarily and predictably block conduction along an axon. The neural impulses are blocked because local anaesthetics inhibit the conformational change needed to activate the Na^+ channel, allowing Na^+ to reenter the cell, causing depolarization.[51] Local anaesthetics also bind to ion channels on other tissues with excitable membranes, which may result in toxicity.

The useful local anaesthetics are mostly weakly basic tertiary amines, with an amine group connected to an aromatic ring via either an ester or an amide linkage. The classification of local anaesthetics into those containing ester or amide linkages is important primarily in differentiating their mode of metabolism. Drugs with an ester linkage (e.g. cocaine, procaine, tetracaine, chloroprocaine) are metabolised by ester hydrolysis (especially by pseudocholinesterase), while those with an amide link (e.g. lignocaine, mepivacaine, prilocaine, bupivacaine, etidocaine, ropivacaine) are degraded mainly by liver microsomal enzymes.

While local anaesthetics are produced as their salt with a strong acid, in aqueous solution this ionises to exist in reversible equilibrium with a weak, unionised, base form. As the unionised form of the local anaesthetic can most readily traverse lipid membranes to reach the ion channel at the site of action, a lower pKa, a higher pH in solution, and greater lipid solubility are all associated with a more rapid onset of action. Alkalinizing local anaesthetic solutions will increase the proportion of free base available and increase the speed of onset. As the free base form is less soluble, increasing the pH of some local anaesthetics (e.g. bupivacaine) may result in precipitation.

The most common use of local anaesthetics in association with intravenous (and inhaled) anaesthetics is to provide supplemental analgesia for postoperative pain relief, but also to reduce the transmission of noxious stimuli during surgery and thereby reduce the requirements for systemic analgesia and anaesthesia. For this purpose, local anaesthetics may be administered by local infiltration or used for peripheral or central nerve blocks. Because of its long duration of action, bupivacaine is the drug most commonly used for this purpose; where speed of onset is more important, however, lignocaine may be a better choice. Local anaesthetic drugs may also be administered intravenously and it is this form of adjunctive use which will be considered here.

Intravenous regional anaesthesia (Bier's block)

Regional anaesthesia can be produced by vascularly isolating a limb, emptying the venous system with a compression bandage, and injecting local anaesthetics intravenously. This technique was first described by August Bier in 1908 and is usually known as a Bier block. In fact, Bier never used exsanguination, instead injecting procaine between two tourniquets. The technique did not become popular until 1963, when Mackinnon Holmes used lignocaine applied to an exsanguinated arm with a single cuff.[52] The onset of regional anaesthesia is rapid, due to delivery of local anaesthetic to cutaneous nerve endings and small nerve branches.[53] Local anaesthetic molecules also travel through the blood vessels supplying the larger nerve trunks, providing deeper analgesia. Diffusion of local anaes-thetic past the isolating tourniquet (either from faulty equipment or too vigorous injection) as well as passage via vessels not compressed by the tourniquet (in and between bones) can allow dangerously high systemic concentrations of local anaesthetic to occur with associated toxicity. In the UK, prilocaine is the drug of choice for iv regional anaesthesia because of its relatively high therapeutic index. In contrast, the relative cardiovascular toxicity of bupivacaine makes it a poor choice for this purpose.

Systemic therapeutic effects of local anaesthetics

Local anaesthetics can elevate pain thresholds and may produce analgesia when given intravenously in chronic and ischaemic pain.[54] Intravenous local anaesthetics have also been used to supplement general anaesthesia. More commonly, local anaesthetics are systemically administered to control ventricular arrhythmias. The agent most commonly used for this purpose is lignocaine, which has the advantage that it does not depress myocardial contractility or alter sinoatrial and atrioventicular node function. Lignocaine predominantly decreases the slope of phase 4 depolarisation in the His-Purkinje system, thereby increasing the threshold for ventricular fibrillation but without changing the resting membrane potential. Other local anaesthetics also act at ion channels in the heart, although differences in their kinetic interactions with myocardial Na^+ channels result in a different balance of beneficial and toxic effects.

Lignocaine dissociates from cardiac Na^+ channels within about 200 ms which permits the Na^+ channels to recover during diastole, even in the presence of a quite marked tachycardia. In contrast, bupivacaine has a dissociation time of approximately 1400–2000 ms. As a result, lignocaine produces a phasic block, thereby slowing cardiac conduction and acting as an antiarrhythmic, whereas bupivacaine results in tonic inhibition of conduction and encourages the generation of arrhythmias via alternative pathways. Lignocaine preferentially blocks Na^+ channels in tissues with longer action potentials (e.g. Purkinje fibres) and therefore has a greater effect on ventricular arrhythmias than on atrial disturbances which are associated with shorter action potentials.

Toxic effects

Toxicity of local anaesthetics results from high blood levels occurring as a result of either direct iv administration or uptake from peripheral tissues into the bloodstream. The uptake of local anaesthetics depends on the absolute amount injected, as well as the vascularity of the site of administration. Subcutaneous administration results in relatively little vascular uptake, whereas systemic absorption is considerable following intercostal block. Absorption from around the brachial plexus and from the epidural space is intermediate between these two extremes. The use of vasoconstrictors can reduce systemic absorption, although this effect varies with the vascularity of the tissue and also depends to some extent on the local anaesthetic used. Absorption of lignocaine and prilocaine is generally faster compared to bupivacaine. Finally, inadvertent vascular injection obviously has a major influence on systemic absorption, hence the need for careful aspiration prior to injection.

The toxic effects of local anaesthetics are most apparent on the CNS. At low doses (1–5 μg/ml) as used as an antiarrhythmic, lignocaine has anticonvulsant activity although higher levels (4·5–7 μg/ml) lead to cortical irritability and convulsions. Similar effects are observed with other local anaesthetics. The anticonvulsant action of local anaesthetics is not clinically useful, however, as there is a narrow therapeutic margin between beneficial

65

and toxic effects.

The earliest signs and symptoms of neurotoxicity are agitation, light-headedness, dizziness, circumoral paraesthesia, visual or auditory disturbances, dysarthria, confusion, and muscle tremors. Tonic-clonic seizures may occur with higher blood concentrations. This spectrum of CNS effects is a result of block of inhibitory neurons followed by disinhibition of excitatory neurons. The likelihood of CNS toxicity can also be influenced by levels of oxygenation, acid–base balance, and the presence of other drugs able to modify seizure threshold. Hyperventilation is a useful measure to reduce CNS toxicity as it increases cerebral oxygenation, reduces cerebral excitability from CO_2 and decreases cerebral blood flow, thereby reducing delivery of local anaesthetic to the brain. In addition, barbiturates, propofol, and benzodiazepines are all effective treatments for local anaesthetic induced seizures.

Local anaesthetics also produce cardiovascular toxicity, although this generally requires higher blood concentrations than those associated with CNS toxicity and is therefore only observed following the rapid iv injection of large doses or when CNS effects are masked by general anaesthesia. A variety of cardiac or peripheral vascular effects may be observed, including ventricular arrhythmias, bradycardia, hypotension, and cardiovascular collapse.

Bupivacaine and, to a lesser extent, etidocaine appear to be associated with a greater degree of CVS toxicity compared to other local anaesthetics and can cause ventricular arrhythmias and fibrillation after iv administration. This is probably due to the longer dissociation time from cardiac Na^+ channels associated with these drugs, producing tonic conduction block. Hypercarbia, acidosis, and hypoxaemia also potentiate the cardiovascular toxicity of bupivacaine.

There is evidence that the cardiac sodium channel is stereospecific. Bupivacaine exists as a racemic mixture and it has been shown that the proarrhythmogenicity of $R(+)$ bupivacaine is several times greater than that of the $S(-)$ enantiomer. This finding may explain the decreased cardiotoxicity of ropivacaine compared to bupivacaine, as ropivacaine is available as a pure $S(-)$ enantiomer. There is also some commercial interest in developing a pure $S(-)$ form of bupivacaine.

In summary, local anaesthetics have a limited role as iv drugs, mainly in the treatment of arrhythmias and for producing iv regional anaesthesia. Topical, local, and regional application of local anaesthetics is nevertheless important in modern anaesthetic practice, enhancing the balanced approach (thereby reducing opioid and anaesthetic doses) and providing prolonged postperative analgesia. Even when local anaesthetics are not directly injected into the bloodstream, vascular uptake may occur and significant blood levels may be achieved so that knowledge of systemic effects and toxicity is important to the anaesthetist.

Other adjuvant drugs

α_2 agonists

The α_2-adrenergic agonists have had a place in veterinary anaesthesia for some time, although they are still considered experimental in humans. Activation of α_2 receptors inhibits adenylate cyclase, reduces cAMP and protein kinase, and alters regulatory proteins to reduce neuronal firing and inhibit neurotransmitter release. The two drugs investigated most extensively in humans are clonidine and dexmedetomidine.

Clonidine is a partial agonist for α_2 receptors. It is rapidly absorbed after oral administration with peak levels reached after 60–90 min and can also be administered from a transdermal patch, although peak levels may take two days to be achieved by this route. Clonidine is relatively long lasting, with hepatic metabolism and renal excretion accounting almost equally for its elimination.

Dexmedetomidine is a full agonist at the α_2 receptor and is more potent and considerably more selective than clonidine.

Use of α_2 agonists in anaesthetic practice   One potential use for the α_2 agonists is in premedication. Clonidine (e.g. 0·3 mg) produces sedation and has an anxiolytic effect comparable to that achieved with the benzodiazepines. This effect occurs relatively rapidly, irrespective of whether clonidine is administered orally or sublingually, allowing its use under a wide variety of circumstances. The α_2 agonists also have an antisialogogue action. Although this property was once considered desirable in a premedicant, it is now regarded as unnecessary by most anaesthetists and unpleasant by most patients. The α_2 agonists also have potent MAC reducing effects, both for iv and inhalational anaesthetics. This property will also be maximally beneficial if the drugs are given preoperatively. Clonidine can reduce the MAC of halothane by approximately 50%, while it reduces the induction dose of iv hypnotics and also produces a 40–45% reduction in opioid requirements. Dexmedetomidine is even more effective in this respect and is reported to reduce the MAC of halothane by 95% in animals.[55] Although these drugs are effective in reducing the requirements for other anaesthetics in humans, they are not capable of producing an anaesthetic state on their own.

The α_2 agonists have potent sympatholytic effects, which may be of particular benefit to patients with coronary artery disease and hypertension. Unfortunately, the extension of these otherwise useful properties often leads to the development of severe bradycardia and/or hypotension. Although bradycardia can be prevented or treated by anticholinergic drugs (e.g. atropine, glycopyrrolate), this may result in an unstable or unpredictable heart rate, which may be undesirable in the presence of CVS disease. To date, there are few data to suggest a more (or less) favourable outcome for patients with severe cardiovascular disease who receive perioperative α_2

agonist drugs compared with those who do not.

The α_2 agonists can also be administered to provide postoperative analgesia. In most cases, these drugs do not appear to be sufficiently efficacious to be used as the sole analgesic agent, although they can prolong analgesia and reduce opioid requirements, which may reduce opioid related side effects, especially respiratory depression. As α_2 agonists have potent sedative effects, their use for postoperative analgesia may delay awakening and later recovery, while the occurrence of bradycardia may again be problematic. The availability of a specific α_2 antagonist (atipamezole) may, however, permit improved recovery and early resolution of adverse effects following α_2 agonists.

In summary, the α_2 drugs have potent sedative, anxiolytic, analgesic, MAC reducing, and cardiovascular stabilising properties. They may prove useful as premedicants, especially in patients with preexisting cardiovascular pathology. Problems remain, however, from extensions of these effects causing toxicity. Residual sedation can delay recovery, while lowering of heart rate may progress to bradycardia requiring rescue medication. Further work is clearly required to determine the optimal place (if any) of these interesting drugs, as well as to critically examine their cost effectiveness and their effect on clinical outcome.

β blockers

The use of β-receptor antagonist drugs can prevent the acute cardiovascular and other somatic manifestations of noxious stimuli, without producing analgesia. During arthroscopic surgery under propofol anaesthesia, the short acting β blocker esmolol provided similar attenuation of the cardiovascular response to surgical stimuli compared to alfentanil.[56] Although β blockers will modify cardiovascular responses to pain, they do not provide analgesia, although they may help to prevent serious cardiovascular disturbances in patients with hypertension. Great care is required not to mask signs of inadequate anaesthesia by the use of β blockers, however, as this may result in awareness associated with considerable pain.

Calcium channel antagonists

Although the calcium channel antagonists are not a routine component of TIVA, they can be used to provide acute control of hypertensive episodes and may also be beneficial in treating acute myocardial ischaemia. These agents may be administered intravenously; however, sublingual delivery also results in rapid absorption.

Muscle relaxants

Muscle relaxants were first used in the 16th century by natives of the Amazon region as arrow poisons for use in hunting. The active ingredient was later found to be curare and it was established in 1850 that this worked at the neuromuscular junction, with no effect on muscles or nerves. Griffith and Johnson are credited with the first use of curare in anaesthesia in 1942,[57] although its use was previously described in a German publication of 1912. Early use of oxygen, N_2O, large doses of muscle relaxants, and hyperventilation (the so-called "Liverpool technique") was associated with a high incidence of intraoperative awareness. Smaller amounts of muscle relaxant are now used to provide adequate relaxation of muscles for surgical access and control of ventilation, while analgesia and hypnosis are also provided by volatile anaesthetics or specific iv drugs. Nevertheless, the incidence of awareness is still higher when muscle relaxant drugs are used compared with when they are not (see chapter 5).

A range of muscle relaxants are currently in clinical use. These agents differ from each other primarily in their speed of onset, their duration of effect, and their associated side effects (table 3.5). Muscle relaxants can also be subdivided into depolarising agents (which act like acetylcholine and stimulate muscles before causing relaxation) and non-depolarising agents (which are competitive antagonists for acetylcholine). The depolarising agents are associated with significantly more side effects and only suxamethonium remains in use, because it has useful properties which have not yet been matched by non-depolarising drugs.

Suxamethonium

Suxamethonium is composed of two acetylcholine molecules linked together via their acetyl groups. Suxamethonium attaches to the acetylcholine receptor, opening the ion channel and causing depolarisation. Unlike acetylcholine, suxamethonium does not dissociate from the receptor immediately, causing a period of relaxation. Most of the side effects of suxamethonium result from depolarisation of neuromuscular junction receptors (e.g. fasciculations, K^+ release) or muscarinic receptors (e.g. bradycardia). The short duration of action of suxamethonium is due to its rapid metabolism by plasma cholinesterase (butyrylcholinesterase), producing succinylmonocholine and ultimately succinic acid and choline. Abnormalities in plasma cholinesterase activity can lead to prolonged block with suxamethonium. The duration of effect is usually moderately increased with acquired deficiencies (e.g. liver disease, plasmapheresis), but may be prolonged to several hours by genetic abnormalities which occur as commonly as once in every 20 000 people. One major advantage of suxamethonium is a rapid onset of profound muscle relaxation, making it ideal for use in emergency cases with full stomachs. A second advantage is a predictably short duration of action (in the absence of cholinesterase deficiencies), making it useful where spontaneous ventilation is required and providing a degree of safety in the event of failed intubation. Because suxamethonium is associated with a number of undesirable side effects

69

Table 3.5 Major pharmacokinetic and pharmacodynamic parameters for currently available muscle relaxants

Drug	ED_{95} (μg/kg)	Usual dose (mg/kg)	Onset (min)	Duration (min)	Clearance (ml/kg/min)	CVS effects	Other effects
Suxamethonium	300	1*	1	4–10	unknown	Bradycardia	See table 3.6
Atracurium	200	0·6*	2	34–45	5·5	Hypotension	Hofmann
Cis-atracurium	50	0·15*	2–3	60–90	5	None	Hofmann
Doxacurium	25	0·05	4	100	2·5	None	
Mivacurium	80	0·15	2	20	4·2	Hypotension	Genetic variability
Pancuronium	50	0·1	2	80–100	1–2	Tachycardia	Renal failure prolongs
Pipecuronium	50	0·1	3	60–120	2·4	None	Renal failure prolongs
Rocuronium	300	0·6	1	30–40	4	Mild tachycardia	Liver failure prolongs
Vecuronium	50	0·1	2·5	25–30	3–4·5	None	
ORG 9487	1150 (ED_{90})	?1·5	1·4	8	8·5	Unknown	Unknown

* Greater than two times ED_{95}

Table 3.6   Problems associated with suxamethonium

Fasciculations
  Muscle pains
  Increased intracranial, intraocular, and intragastric pressure
Potassium release
  Production of arrhythmias and/or cardiac arrest
  More severe with denervation (e.g. burns, paraplegia, neuromuscular disease) (baseline K^+
    may already be raised in renal failure)
Cardiovascular
  Bradycardia and/or asystole (especially with repeat dose)
Muscle diseases
  Potent trigger to malignant hyperpyrexia
  Exaggerated K^+ response in some myopathies
Prolonged duration
  Genetic cholinesterase abnormalities
  Acquired cholinesterase deficiencies
  Type II block with prolonged administration

(table 3.6), its use is now largely confined to those situations where it conveys a distinct advantage over the alternatives.

Non-depolarising relaxants

Structurally, the non-depolarising muscle relaxants may be divided into the benzylisoquinolinium group and the steroid group. The benzylisoquinoliniums are more prone to release histamine, with the possibility of cardiovascular effects. When evaluating muscle relaxant drugs, a number of parameters are usually quoted. The potency is defined by the term ED_{95}, which is the average dose required to produce 95% depression of the adductor policis muscle twitch. The usual intubating dose is twice ED_{95}, although for some drugs with a slow onset of action, it is common to administer three times ED_{95}. The onset time is measured from drug administration until peak effect, although tracheal intubation may be possible somewhat earlier than this endpoint. For any given drug, a larger dose results in a more rapid attainment of a given effect, although duration will also be prolonged. Between drugs, there appears to be an inverse correlation between potency and speed of onset, with the most rapidly acting drugs also being the least potent. The duration of a muscle relaxant is usually given as the time required for a 25% recovery of twitch height. This broadly correlates to the time at which a supplemental dose will be required for surgical relaxation, although this also depends on many other factors.

Most modern non-depolarising muscle relaxants have a reasonably rapid clearance and are non-cumulative. This means that the nth increment lasts for as long as the first. With some of the earlier relaxants, as well as in the presence of renal and/or hepatic disease, duration of effect may be prolonged. Atracurium and cis-atracurium are less susceptible to prolongation of their effect by organ dysfunction because they do not rely on the liver

71

or kidney for their metabolism or elimination. Instead, these drugs degrade spontaneously in the plasma, a process which is known as Hofmann elimination. Monitoring of neuromuscular block can provide useful information on duration of effect and recovery and allows redosing to be practised in a logical manner. Spontaneous recovery to a train of four (TOF) ratio of $\geqslant 70\%$ is sometimes quoted for shorter duration muscle relaxants. This is the endpoint which best correlates with safe removal of the tracheal tube. For most non-depolarising relaxants, spontaneous recovery occurs too slowly to be used frequently and "reversal" drugs are frequently administered (see chapter 3).

The key pharmacokinetic and pharmacodynamic properties of the non-depolarising muscle relaxants are conveniently shown in table 3.5. Additional points are briefly outlined below.

Atracurium and cis-atracurium

Although atracurium is metabolised by the liver and excreted by the kidney, it also undergoes spontaneous degradation into inactive components by a process of Hofmann elimination. This process preferentially occurs at body temperature and pH, making atracurium relatively stable in an acid solution at low temperature. The Hofmann pathway provides an alternative route of elimination even in the absence of hepatic and/or renal function. The major disadvantage of atracurium is a tendency to histamine release, overcome by cis-atracurium, one of ten optical isomers of atracurium. Cis-atracurium does not release histamine and is associated with cardiovascular stability. It is more potent than atracurium and therefore has a slower onset. This is partially offset by the use of a three times ED_{95} dose, although this results in a longer duration. Cis-atracurium also undergoes Hofmann elimination.

Mivacurium

Mivacurium is the shortest duration non-depolarising muscle relaxant currently available. Like suxamethonium, its effect is terminated by pseudocholinesterase and the possibility of a prolonged effect exists in individuals with abnormal levels of this enzyme. Mivacurium is also associated with a considerable degree of histamine release which can result in severe cardiovascular depression. This effect can be reduced by the use of a low dose, administered slowly, although this benefit is offset by a considerably slower onset and shortened duration of effect.

Pancuronium

Pancuronium was the first synthetic steroid muscle relaxant. It has some vagolytic effects resulting in tachycardia, increased blood pressure, and cardiac output. It is also extensively excreted in urine and may accumulate in renal failure. Pancuronium is seldom used because of its long duration and cardiovascular side effects. It is sometimes still used in cardiac anaesthesia, however, where its vagolytic effects can compensate for the bradycardia often produced by high dose opioids.

Vecuronium

Vecuronium is structurally related to pancuronium but is associated with excellent cardiovascular stability and an intermediate duration. As vecuronium undergoes both renal excretion and hepatic metabolism, it is less affected by organ dysfunction, although not to the same degree as atracurium.

Rocuronium

Rocuronium is very similar to vecuronium except for a faster onset of effect. Tracheal intubating conditions at one minute after relaxant administration have been shown to be comparable between rocuronium and suxamethonium.[58] Rocuronium produces a mild tachycardia at high dose (although not as significant as with pancuronium) and is also more likely to accumulate in hepatic failure than vecuronium.

Doxacurium and pipecuronium

These two agents are both very long acting muscle relaxants (comparable to pancuronium) but without significant cardiovascular side effects. With a general move towards the use of multiple doses (or infusions) of short acting muscle relaxants, there is very little clinical use of these agents in the United States. They are not currently available in the United Kingdom.

Future developments

There has long been a desire to develop a non-depolarising muscle relaxant with both the rapid onset of action and short duration of effect associated with suxamethonium. To date, rapid onset (rocuronium) and (relatively) short duration (mivacurium) have been achieved individually, but not combined in the same drug. A number of "non-depolarising suxamethonium replacement" compounds have undergone animal and early clinical trials. Currently, the most promising agent is ORG 9487. This has the low potency associated with fast onset, with an ED_{90} value of $1 \cdot 15$ mg/kg. The average onset time after $1 \cdot 5$ mg/kg $(1 \cdot 3 \times ED_{90})$ was 83 s, only slightly longer than that of suxamethonium (67 s), and tracheal intubating conditions at one minute were similar with either relaxant.[59] Although spontaneous recovery to a TOF ratio of $\geqslant 70\%$ required 24 min, this could be reduced to only $11 \cdot 6$ min if neostigmine was administered within two minutes of the initial relaxant dose.[59] This unusual strategy might prove useful in the event of a "failed intubation". Unlike suxamethonium or mivacurium, recovery from ORG 9487 is not dependent on cholinesterase activity. Nevertheless, this drug is still inferior to suxamethonium in terms of duration of effect and it remains to be seen whether the large dose required (because of low potency) will be prohibitively expensive or associated with significant side effects.

In summary, the muscle relaxants are a valuable component of modern balanced and total intravenous anaesthesia. Most of the currently available drugs have highly specific actions with minimal side effects (especially vecuronium and cis-atracurium). Nevertheless, muscle relaxants do introduce specific problems, including variability in duration of effect, accumulation in some disease states, and inadequate reversal of effects. Some muscle relaxants also add their own side effects (e.g. histamine release), although this is less common with newer drugs. The muscle relaxants are unique in that their effects can be directly and accurately monitored and it is somewhat surprising that neuromuscular monitoring is not more commonly employed. Finally, it must be remembered that the use of muscle relaxant drugs abolishes a useful sign of inadequate anaesthesia and increases the incidence of awareness. For this reason, muscle relaxants should only be administered where they are really necessary and the minimum dose necessary should be used.

Intravenous antagonist drugs

Opioid antagonists

Naloxone is a specific opioid antagonist, capable of reversing all the effects of opioids, therapeutic and adverse. It acts within 1–2 min of intravenous administration but has a short duration of effect. The duration of action of naloxone is usually shorter than that of the opioid being antagonised, meaning that adverse events may recur and the dose of naloxone may need to be repeated. As naloxone reverses all opioid effects, it should be administered very slowly and carefully until the adverse event requiring therapy is abolished. When used in this way, a degree of analgesia may remain after naloxone's use. An alternative approach is to use a pure respiratory stimulant such as doxapram, which will frequently overcome opioid induced ventilatory depression, while having no effect on analgesia. Careful titration of the initial opioid therapy to the desired clinical effect can also reduce the need for treatment with antagonists.

Nalmephene is another opioid antagonist which has recently become available. It is substantially longer lasting than naloxone and should reduce the likelihood of a recurrence of opioid side effects ("renarcotisation"). Nalmephene is effective in a dose of 0·25 μg/kg, repeated at 2–3 min intervals until an optimal effect is achieved. Like naloxone, nalmephene reverses all the opioid effects, beneficial and harmful. Naltrexone is another long acting opioid antagonist. It can also be given by mouth and has been used via this route to reduce opioid induced pruritus following epidural opioids. Some of the pharmacokinetic parameters for the opioid antagonists are summarised in table 3.4.

Benzodiazepine antagonists

Flumazenil is a competitive benzodiazepine receptor antagonist, able to reverse all the behavioural, neurological, and electrophysiological effects of benzodiazepine agonists. It is soluble in acidic aqueous solutions and, like other benzodiazepines, is highly protein bound. Flumazenil is rapidly cleared from plasma (5–20 ml/kg/min) secondary to rapid hepatic metabolism. It has a $T_{1/2}\beta$ of 0·7–1·3 h and a Vd_{ss} of 0·6–1·6 l/kg.

Flumazenil has minimal intrinsic CNS, CVS or respiratory effects. Doses of 0·1–0·2 mg will partially antagonise benzodiazepine effects, while 0·4–1·0 mg is required for complete antagonism (assuming usual sedative doses of benzodiazepines have been used). Flumazenil may be useful in the diagnosis of prolonged sedation in the ICU. It can also hasten recovery when benzodiazepines are used for conscious sedation. As the plasma clearance of flumazenil is greater than that of midazolam (and other benzodiazepines) the possibility of resedation exists when a single dose of flumazenil is used to reverse sedation resulting from a large dose (or an infusion) of midazolam.[60] This resedation is less likely if the initial midazolam dose was the minimal effective amount, however (fig 3.3).[61]

Muscle relaxant antagonists

It is common practice to antagonise muscle relaxants. This is because while clinically adequate muscle relaxation declines relatively rapidly, return of full neuromuscular power may take a much longer time. This is because of the considerable reserve of neuromuscular junctional receptors which exist on normal muscle. Muscle power sufficient for movements and even ventilation can be attained even in the presence of moderate neuromuscular block. The ability to sustain a tetanic contraction (as is needed for most physiological movements) or to produce a cough to protect the airway requires substantially more power and is only possible when most neuromuscular junctions are functioning normally. Antagonist drugs are therefore routinely administered except when neuromuscular blocking drugs with very brief duration of action (e.g. suxamethonium, mivacurium) have been used or when a long period has elapsed since the last dose of relaxant and the patient is able to sustain a physiological tetanus (e.g. a five second head lift) or has a TOF ratio of 70% or more.

The muscle relaxant antagonists are anticholinesterases which inhibit the hydrolysis of acetylcholine (at all cholinergic synapses). Acetylcholine is therefore present at the synapse for longer, allowing it to compete more favourably with the muscle relaxant for the neuromuscular receptor. As

75

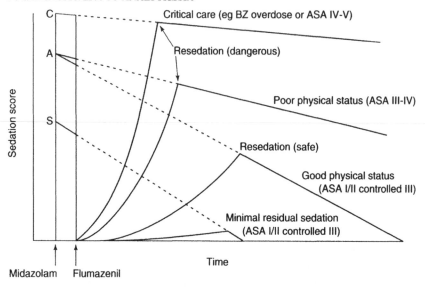

Fig 3.3   Clinical interaction between midazolam and flumazenil in different clinical situations. C Critically ill patient; A Anaesthetic dose of midazolam in patients with delayed elimination (upper line) or normal elimination (lower line); S Sedation dose of midazolam; BZ Benzodiazepine. Dotted line indicates sedation score in absence of flumazenil. Reproduced with permission[61]

anticholinesterases are active at all cholinergic synapses, the effects of acetylcholine at synapses in the autonomic nervous system will also be potentiated. For these reasons, anticholinesterases are usually administered along with an anticholinergic such as atropine or glycopyrrolate, which will act at all cholinergic synapses *except* the neuromuscular junction. The anticholinesterases used clinically are reversible and have a duration of effect similar to or slightly longer than that of the relaxants they antagonise. The two most commonly used anticholinesterases are neostigmine and edrophonium. Neostigmine is usually administered in a dose of 35 μg/kg (with atropine 10–20 μg/kg) and reaches peak effect in 5–7 min, provided a degree of spontaneous recovery from the muscle relaxant has already occurred. For a more profound block, a larger dose may be necessary, although recovery of adequate neuromuscular function is likely to be delayed. Edrophonium (0·5–1 mg/kg) has a faster onset compared to neostigmine and is also of shorter duration. It is suitable for use provided that an intermediate duration muscle relaxant has been used. With longer lasting relaxants, there is the possibility of a recurrence of muscle weakness after the effects of edrophonium wear off.

Excessive doses of anticholinesterases can produce a depolarising-like neuromuscular block, although this is much less common than inadequate reversal of a non-depolarising block. There is also some evidence that the use of anticholinesterases increases the incidence of PONV. Their use has also been associated with a greater rate of breakdown of bowel anastamoses. It would therefore seem logical to avoid the use of muscle relaxant antagonists wherever possible, an aim best achieved by the use of low doses of very short acting muscle relaxants and careful monitoring of their effect.

Summary

Many intravenous hypnotic agents have come and gone over the years. Of all those, propofol is currently by far the most widely used, although it is possible that reformulated etomidate and (possibly) optically pure ketamine may become more important in the future. Propofol has become so widely employed because its short duration of effect makes it easy to use in brief procedures where rapid recovery is important and in longer cases where rapid response to reduced drug delivery improves control of anaesthetic depth. As a maintenance anaesthetic as part of a balanced technique, infusion rates of 75–200 µg/kg/min (or a "target" concentration of 3–7 µg/ml) are usually required, while higher levels of 100–300 µg/kg/min (6–10 µg/ml) will be required if propofol is used alone. Lower doses of propofol can also be used for sedation and it has proved just as valuable (if not more so) in this role as it has for general anaesthesia. Typical sedative infusion rates for propofol are 25–75 µg/kg/min (0·5–1 µg/ml).

It is usually necessary to supplement iv anaesthetics with opioid analgesics. Until recently, alfentanil (or sufentanil where it is available) was the most commonly used opioid. Because of its short duration of action, alfentanil is usually given by infusion. To supplement propofol anaesthesia, a loading dose of 25–50 µg/kg followed by an infusion of 0·5–2 µg/kg/min (equivalent to a plasma concentration of 100–200 ng/ml) is usually sufficient. Remifentanil may soon become the opioid of choice to supplement propofol anaesthesia. Infusion rates of 0·25–0·5 µg/kg/min are suitable for most procedures, although the dose can easily be increased without seriously delaying recovery. Where analgesia is required rapidly (e.g. to blunt the response to intubation), a loading dose of remifentanil 0·25–0·5 µg/kg may be given. Alternatively, adequate analgesia is established within only a few minutes of commencing an infusion. Remifentanil may also have a place in conscious sedation, especially for procedures with a moderate degree of intraoperative pain. Infusion rates of 0·1 µg/kg/min provide adequate "sedation" without significant respiratory depression. Care should also be taken with the use of non-opioid forms of analgesia, with local anaesthetic instillation and NSAIDs being used wherever possible to reduce the requirements for opioids and the occurrence of side effects and to improve the quality of analgesia.

Muscle relaxants may be required as part of a TIVA or balanced iv anaesthetic. A wide choice of agents is now available and modern muscle relaxants are generally free of side effects and their duration of effect is relatively independent of major organ function. The choice of agent will depend primarily on the required duration of action. The newer drugs are shorter acting or have faster onset, and it is hoped that the future will see both of these properties combined in a single non-depolarising muscle relaxant.

Although specific antagonists exist for benzodiazepines, opioids, and the muscle relaxants, it is only the latter group which are used routinely. This is primarily because the available antagonists are significantly shorter lasting than their agonist counterparts, so that their use to "reverse" excessive sedation or respiratory depression may induce a dangerous false sense of security, with problems recurring later when patients are less well supervised. In addition, the use of antagonists introduces further potential side effects and as shorter acting drugs are developed (e.g. mivacurium, remifentanil), antagonists are likely to be used even less.

1 Borgeat A, Wilder-Smith OHG, Jallon P, Suter PM. Propofol in the management of refractory status epilepticus: a case report. *Intens Care Med* 1994;20:148–9.
2 Reddy RV, Moorthy SS, Dierdorf SF, Deitch RD Jr, Link L. Excitatory effects and electroencephalographic correlation of etomidate, thiopental, methohexital, and propofol. *Anesth Analg* 1993;77:1008–11.
3 Grounds RM, Twigley AJ, Carli F, Whitwam JG, Morgan M. The haemodynamic effects of intravenous induction. Comparison of the effects of thiopentone and propofol. *Anaesthesia* 1985;40:735–40.
4 Roberts FL, Dixon J, Lewis GTR, Tackley RM, Prys-Roberts C. Induction and maintenance of propofol anaesthesia. A manual infusion scheme. *Anaesthesia* 1988;43(supplement):14–7.
5 Haessler R, Madler C, Klasing S, Schwender D, Peter K. Propofol/fentanyl versus etomidate fentanyl for the induction of anesthesia in patients with aortic insufficiency and coronary artery disease. *J Cardiothorac Vasc Anesth* 1992;6:173–80.
6 Underwood SM, Davies SW, Feneck RO, Walesby RK. Anaesthesia for myocardial revascularisation: a comparison of fentanyl/propofol with fentanyl/enflurane. *Anaesthesia* 1992;47:939–45.
7 Hall RI, Murphy JT, Landymore R, *et al.* Myocardial metabolic changes during propofol anesthesia for cardiac surgery in patients with reduced ventricular function. *Anesth Analg* 1993;77:680–9.
8 Chong JL, Grebenik C, Sinclair M, *et al.* The effect of a cardiac surgical recovery area on the timing of extubation. *J Cardiothorac Vasc Anesth* 1993;7:137–41.
9 Robertson WR, Reader SCJ, Davison B, *et al.* On the biopotency and site of action of drugs affecting endocrine tissue with special reference to the anti-steroidogenic effect of anaesthetic agents. *Postgrad Med J* 1985;61(supplement 3):145–51.
10 Aitkenhead AR, Pepperman ML, Willatts SM, *et al.* Comparison of propofol and midazolam for sedation in critically ill patients. Lancet 1989;ii:704–9.
11 Fredman B, d'Etienne J, Smith I, Husain MM, White PF. Anesthesia for electroconvulsive therapy: effects of propofol and methohexital on seizure activity and recovery. *Anesth Analg* 1994;79:75–9.
12 McKenzie AJ, Couchman KG, Pollock N. Propofol is a safe anaesthetic agent in malignant hyperthermia susceptible patients. *Anaesth Intens Care* 1992;20:165–8.
13 Borgeat A, Wilder-Smith OHG, Suter PM. The nonhypnotic therapeutic applications of propofol. *Anesthesiology* 1994;80:642–56.
14 DiFlorio T. Is propofol a dopamine antagonist? (letter). *Anesth Analg* 1993;77:200–1.

15 Smith I, White PF, Nathanson M, Gouldson R. Propofol: an update on its clinical use. *Anesthesiology* 1994;**81**:1005–43.
16 Borgeat A, Wilder-Smith OHG, Saiah M, Rifat K. Subhypnotic doses of propofol possess direct antiemetic properties. *Anesth Analg* 1992;**74**:539–41.
17 Klement W, Arndt JO. Pain on injection of propofol: effects of concentration and diluent. *Br J Anaesth* 1991;**67**:281–4.
18 Corssen G, Domino EF. Dissociative anesthesia: further pharmacologic studies and first clinical experience with the phencyclidine derivative CI-581. *Anesth Analg* 1966;**42**:29–40.
19 White PF, Ham J, Way WL, Trevor AJ. Pharmacology of ketamine isomers in surgical patients. *Anesthesiology* 1980;**52**:231–9.
20 Clements JA, Nimmo WS. The pharmacokinetics and analgesic effect of ketamine in man. *Br J Anaesth* 1981;**53**:27–30.
21 White PF, Schüttler J, Shafer A, *et al.* Comparative pharmacology of the ketamine isomers. Studies in volunteers. *Br J Anaesth* 1985;**57**:197–203.
22 Chodoff P. Evidence for central adrenergic action of ketamine. *Anesth Analg* 1972;**51**:247–50.
23 Coppel DL, Bovill JG, Dundee JW. The taming of ketamine. *Anaesthesia* 1973;**28**:293–6.
24 Hatano S, Keane DM, Boggs RE, El-Naggar MA, Sadove MS. Diazepam-ketamine anaesthesia for open heart surgery. A "micro-mini" drip administration technique. *Can Anaesth Soc J* 1976;**23**:648–55.
25 Gutzke GE, Shah K, Glisson SN, Griesemer R, Rao TLK. Sufentanil or ketamine: Induction in cardiomyopathy patients. *Anesthesiology* 1987;**67**:A64.
26 Marietta MP, Way WL, Castagnoli N, Trevor AJ. On the pharmacology of the ketamine enantiomorphs in the rat. *J Pharmacol Exp Ther* 1977;**202**:157–65.
27 Ryder S, Way WL. Comparative pharmacology of the optical isomers of ketamine in mice. *Eur J Pharmacol* 1978;**49**:15–23.
28 van Hamme MJ, Ghonheim MM, Ambre JJ. Pharmacokinetics of etomidate, a new intravenous anesthetic. *Anesthesiology* 1978;**49**:274.
29 Renou AM, Vernhiet J, Macrez P, *et al.* Cerebral blood flow and metabolism during etomidate anaesthesia in man. *Br J Anaesth* 1978;**50**:1047.
30 Ledingham IM, Watt I. Influence of sedation on mortality in critically ill multiple trauma patients (letter). *Lancet* 1983;**1**:1270.
31 Wagner RL, White PF, Kan PB, Rosenthal MH, Feldman D. Inhibition of adrenal steroidogenesis by the anesthetic etomidate. *NEJM* 1984;**310**:1415–21.
32 Doenicke A, Roizen MF, Nebauer AE, *et al.* A comparison of two formulations for etomidate, 2-hydroxypropyl-β-cyclodextrin (HPCD) and propylene glycol. *Anesth Analg* 1994;**79**:933–9.
33 Doenicke A, Kugler A, Vollmann N, Suttmann H, Taeger K. Etomidate with a new solubilizer. Clinical and experimental investigations on venous tolerance and bio-availability. *Anaesthetist* 1990;**39**:475–80.
34 Doenicke A, Kugler A, Vollmann N. Venous tolerance to etomidate in lipid emulsion or propylene glycol (hypnomidate). *Can J Anaesth* 1990;**37**:823–4.
35 Montmorency FA, Chen A, Rudel H, Glas WW, Lee LE. Evaluation of cardiovascular and general pharmacologic properties of hydroxydione. *Anesthesiology* 1958;**19**:450–6.
36 Moneret-Vautrin DA, Laxenaire MC, Viry-Babel F. Anaphylaxis caused by anti-Cremophor EL IgG STS antibodies in a case of reaction to Althesin. *Br J Anaesth* 1983;**55**:469–71.
37 Van Hemelrijck J, Muller P, Van Aken H, White PF. Relative potency of eltanolone, propofol, and thiopental for induction of anesthesia. *Anesthesiology* 1994;**80**:36–41.
38 Kallela H, Haasio J, Korttila K. Comparison of eltanolone and propofol in anesthesia for termination of pregnancy. *Anesth Analg* 1994;**79**:512–16.
39 Bailey P, Gerbode F, Garlington L. An anesthetic technique for cardiac surgery which utilizes 100% oxygen as the only inhalant. *Arch Surg* 1958;**76**:437–43.
40 Ling GSF, Spiegel K, Lockhart SH, Pasternak GW. Separation of opioid analgesia from respiratory depression: evidence for different receptor mechanisms. *J Pharmacol Exp Ther* 1985;**232**:149–55.
41 Westmoreland CL, Hoke JF, Sebel PS, Hug CC, Muir KT. Pharmacokinetics of

remifentanil (G187084B) and its major metabolite (G190291) in patients undergoing elective inpatient surgery. *Anesthesiology* 1993;**79**:893–903.

42 Dershwitz M, Randel GI, Rosow CE, *et al.* Initial clinical experience with remifentanil, a new opioid metabolized by esterases. *Anesth Analg* 1995;**81**:619–23.

43 Chauvin M, Lebrault C, Levron JC, Duvaldestin P. Pharmacokinetics of alfentanil in chronic renal failure. *Anesth Analg* 1987;**66**:53–6.

44 Hoke JF, Muir KT, Glass PSA, *et al.* Pharmacokinetics of remifentanil and its metabolite (GI90291) in subjects with renal disease (abstract). *Clin Pharmacol Ther* 1995;**57**:PI55.

45 Mendel P, Fredman B, White PF. Alfentanil suppresses coughing and agitation during emergence from isoflurane anesthesia. *J Clin Anesth* 1995;**7**:114–8.

46 Bjertraes LJ. Hypoxia-induced vasoconstriction in isolated perfused lungs exposed to injectable or inhalation anesthetics. *Acta Anaesthesiol Scand* 1977;**21**:133–47.

47 Rich GF, Schacterle R, Moscicki JC, DiFazio CA. Ketorolac does not decrease the MAC of halothane or depress ventilation in rats. *Anesth Analg* 1992;**75**:99–102.

48 Ding Y, Fredman B, White PF. Use of ketorolac and fentanyl during outpatient gynecologic surgery. *Anesth Analg* 1993;**77**:205–10.

49 Kenny GNC. Ketorolac trometamol – a new non-opiod analgesic. *Br J Anaesth* 1990; **65**:445–7.

50 Dordoni PL, Della Ventura M, Stefanelli A, *et al.* Effect of ketorolac, ketoprofen and nefopam on platelet function. *Anaesthesia* 1994;**49**:1046–9.

51 Butterworth JF, Strichartz GR. Molecular mechanisms of local anesthesia: a review. *Anesthesiology* 1990;**72**:711–34.

52 Calverley RK. Anesthesia as a specialty: past, present, and future. In: Barash PG, Cullen BF, Stoelting RK, eds, *Clinical Anesthesia*. Philadelphia: J. B. Lippincott, 1989:3–33.

53 Raj PP, Garcia CE, Burleson JW, Jenkins MT. The site of action of intravenous regional anesthesia. *Anesth Analg* 1972;**51**:776–86.

54 Kastrup J, Angelo H, Petersen P, Dejgarda A, Hilstead J. Treatment of chronic painful diabetic neuropathy with intravenous lidocaine infusion. *Br Med J* 1986;**292**:173.

55 Segal IS, Vickery RG, Walton JK, Doze VA, Maze M. Dexmedetomidine diminishes halothane anesthetic requirements in rats through a postsynaptic alpha2 adrenergic receptors. *Anesthesiology* 1988;**69**:818–23.

56 Smith I, van Hemelrijck J, White PF. Efficacy of esmolol versus alfentanil as a supplement to propofol-N_2O anesthesia. *Anesth Analg* 1991;**73**:540–6.

57 Griffith HR, Johnson GE. The use of curare in general anesthesia. *Anesthesiology* 1942;**3**:418–20.

58 Pühringer FK, Khueni-Brady KS, Koller J, Mitterschiffthaler G. Evaluation of the endotracheal intubating conditions of rocuronium (ORG 9426) and succinylcholine in outpatient surgery. *Anesth Analg* 1992;**75**:37–40.

59 Wierda JMKH, van den Broek L, Proost JH, Verbaan BW, Hennis PJ. Time course of action and endotracheal intubating conditions of Org 9487, a new short-acting steroidal muscle relaxant: a comparison with succinylcholine. *Anesth Analg* 1993;**77**:579–84.

60 Ghouri AF, Ramirez Ruiz MA, White PF. Effect of flumazenil on recovery after midazolam and propofol sedation. *Anesthesiology* 1994;**81**:333–9.

61 Whitwam JG. Midazolam-flumazenil: an update. *Min Invas Ther* 1995;**4**(supplement 2):31–8.

62 Shafer SL. Advances in propofol pharmacokinetics and pharmacodynamics. *J Clin Anesth* 1993;**5**(supplement 1):14S–21S.

4: Use of intravenous anaesthesia techniques in special patient populations

Introduction

Intravenous anaesthetic techniques are applicable in virtually all patients and surgical procedures. Naturally, every patient and procedure will be subtly different from all the others and so the anaesthetic technique will have to be adapted to the particular circumstances of each individual case. Nevertheless, there are certain groups of patients which present a broadly similar set of problems and challenges and which can conveniently be discussed as a group. In day case surgery, the patients are reasonably healthy and the emphasis is on rapid, clearheaded recovery associated with minimal side effects, including those which would elsewhere be considered "minor". Children differ from adults in their physiology, requiring a different range of drug doses for anaesthetic induction and maintenance. The range of surgical and associated pathology encountered in paediatric practice also differs from that seen in adults, presenting different challenges. Elderly patients also have different responses to anaesthetic drugs than their younger counterparts. In addition, they are more likely to have clinically significant coexisting diseases which may affect their response to anaesthesia and surgery. Critically ill patients obviously represent a high risk population as a result of acute and severe disturbances of physiology, often superimposed on a background of chronic illness. This chapter will consider some of the important aspects in the anaesthetic management of these four special groups of patients.

Day case patients

Because of the need for same-day discharge, the ideal day case anaesthetic must permit a rapid recovery with minimal side effects in addition to the usual requirements for smooth induction and optimum intraoperative conditions. In the early days of day case anaesthesia, methohexitone was a popular iv anaesthetic as recovery from its effects was much more rapid compared to thiopentone. As better anaesthetics have become available, the use of methohexitone has declined, however. Etomidate also enjoyed brief popularity as a day case anaesthetic. Although it is associated with an acceptable rate of recovery, a high incidence of PONV is its main disadvantage in day cases, although its other adverse effects are also problematic. Ketamine is also associated with a number of problems. Even when its hallucinatory properties are "tamed", ketamine still has a slower onset of action and a delayed recovery compared to alternative agents and is therefore rarely used for induction or maintenance of day case anaesthesia. Propofol has rapidly become the day case iv anaesthetic of choice as it fulfils the criteria for a day case anaesthetic better than other currently available agents.

Propofol

Propofol offers many advantages over the other available intravenous induction agents because of its smooth and rapid onset of action, rapid recovery, and minimal side effects.[1] The duration of clinical action of propofol is short and recovery from its effects rapid because of early redistribution and a high metabolic clearance rate. Propofol has been compared with a variety of other drugs as a day case anaesthetic induction agent (table 4.1). Compared to thiopentone, propofol has usually been shown to result in more rapid emergence and/or improved performance in psychomotor testing during the early recovery period, in both adults and children. Use of propofol in place of thiopentone as the induction agent may even result in earlier discharge of day case patients.

In comparison to methohexitone, propofol is associated with greater alertness, improved performance on reaction time testing, and a shorter period of postoperative ataxia. Although recovery times appear similar after induction doses of either propofol or etomidate, propofol is associated with fewer postoperative side effects compared with either etomidate or methohexitone.

Propofol is also superior to other iv maintenance agents for day case anaesthesia (table 4.2). Emergence generally occurs significantly earlier with propofol compared to other intravenous maintenance anaesthetics, with improved recovery becoming more apparent following longer surgical procedures. Differences in recovery may still be apparent 24 h after anaesthesia when propofol is compared with barbiturates. In addition to improvements in emergence and recovery times achieved with propofol, the quality of anaesthesia is usually superior to alternative intravenous maintenance agents. Compared to etomidate, intravenous anaesthesia with propofol is more stable and easier to conduct, while propofol produces better muscle relaxation and less hiccuping than either thiopentone or methohexitone, resulting in improved surgical conditions. A reduced incidence of PONV has also been reported after the use of propofol for

Table 4.1   Comparison of propofol with alternative induction agents for day case anaesthesia

Reference	Comparator	Maintenance	Principal findings*
DeGrood et al., 1987	Thiopentone	Isoflurane	Faster emergence and improved test results
Gupta et al., 1992	Thiopentone	Isoflurane	Improved test results for first 90 min
Chittleborough et al., 1992	Thiopentone	Enflurane	Faster emergence and discharge
Ding et al., 1993	Thiopentone	Enflurane	Faster emergence, recovery times similar
Mackenzie & Grant, 1985	Thiopentone	Enflurane	Greatly improved psychomotor performance
Rolly & Versichelen, 1985	Thiopentone	Halothane/ isoflurane	Faster emergence, later events not reported
Runcie et al., 1993	Thiopentone	Halothane/ isoflurane	Faster emergence, earlier discharge in older children only
Sanders et al., 1989	Thiopentone	Halothane	Similar emergence and recovery
O'Toole et al., 1987	Methohexitone	Isoflurane	Faster emergence, improvements at 20 min
Mackenzie & Grant, 1985	Methohexitone	Enflurane	Improved psychomotor performance
Valanne & Korttila, 1985	Methohexitone	Enflurane	Similar times to orientation and ambulation
DeGrood et al., 1987	Etomidate	Isoflurane	Non-significantly faster recovery
Norton & Dundas, 1990	Midazolam-flumazenil	Isoflurane	Improved psychomotor performance

* Findings are expressed with respect to the propofol group
Modified with permission from[1]

Table 4.2   Comparison of propofol with alternative intravenous techniques for day case anaesthesia

Reference	Administration	Comparator	Principal findings*
DeGrood et al., 1987	FRI	Etomidate	Faster and more predictable recovery
Heath et al., 1988	IB	Etomidate	Faster emergence, smoother induction
Cade et al., 1991	IB	Methohexitone	Faster recovery to ambulation
Cundy & Arunasalam, 1985	IB	Methohexitone	Improved "quality" of anaesthesia, less drowsy
Doze et al., 1986	VRI	Methohexitone	Earlier orientation and ambulation
Heath et al., 1988	IB	Methohexitone	Similar recovery times
Jakobsson et al., 1993	IB	Methohexitone	Early recovery not reported, discharge similar
Kay & Healy, 1985	IB	Methohexitone	Faster emergence and psychomotor recovery
Mackenzie & Grant, 1985	VRI	Methohexitone	Faster emergence, smoother anaesthetic
Noble & Ogg, 1985	IB	Methohexitone	Similar emergence and recovery times
Ræder & Misvær, 1988	IB	Methohexitone	Faster emergence, recovery times similar
Sampson et al., 1988	IB	Thiamylal	Faster emergence, later events not reported
Edelist, 1987	IB	Thiopentone	Faster emergence and orientation
Heath et al., 1988	IB	Thiopentone	Faster emergence, recovery times similar
Heath et al., 1990	IB	Thiopentone	Reduced tiredness at 24 h postoperative
Henriksson et al., 1987	IB	Thiopentone	Faster emergence, later events not reported
Jakobsson et al., 1993	IB	Thiopentone	Faster discharge
Johnston et al., 1987	IB	Thiopentone	Faster emergence, later events not reported
Korttila et al., 1992	2 boluses	Thiopentone	Faster emergence and psychomotor recovery
Nielsen et al., 1991	FRI	Thiopentone	Similar emergence and recovery times
Ræder & Misvær, 1988	IB	Thiopentone	Faster emergence and psychomotor recovery
Ryom et al., 1992	IB	Thiopentone	Similar performance in postoperative testing
Sanders et al., 1991	IB	Thiopentone	Faster emergence, improvements at 24 h

VRI Variable rate infusion; FRI Fixed rate infusion; IB Intermittent bolus doses
* Findings are expressed with respect to the propofol group
Modified with permission from[1]

induction and maintenance of anaesthesia compared to other iv anaesthetics. PONV is especially undesirable following day case surgery, not only because of the unpleasantness of these symptoms for the patient but also because it can significantly delay discharge and may necessitate admission to hospital. There is now an increasing body of evidence that propofol possesses distinct antiemetic properties.[2]

Propofol is not completely free of unwanted side effects. It produces more profound hypotension than other iv anaesthetics agents, primarily as a result of peripheral vasodilation, although this phenomenon is likely to be less of a problem in relatively healthy day case patients. Pain on injection is troublesome to day case patients, but can be minimised by the prophylactic administration of lignocaine. Propofol may also improve the mood of patients in the postoperative period, producing a euphoria-like state, which appears to be well received.

How does total or balanced anaesthesia with propofol compare with volatile anaesthetics in day case patients? Such comparisons are difficult because of the problems in ensuring similar depths of anaesthesia with both types of technique. Until an objective, anaesthetic agent independent monitor of anaesthetic depth is developed, the practitioner has to rely on clinical signs. Unfortunately, the relationship between anaesthetic depth and haemodynamic parameters does not appear to be as simple for iv anaesthetics as it is with the inhaled agents (chapter 5).

A number of investigations have shown that induction and maintenance of anaesthesia with propofol results in faster emergence and recovery than induction with thiopentone and maintenance with volatile anaesthetics. This type of study does not separate the effect of the induction agent (propofol versus thiopentone) from that of the maintenance drug (propofol versus inhaled anaesthetic), however. When propofol is used for induction of anaesthesia, followed by either propofol or a volatile agent for maintenance, awakening has usually occurred later after the inhalational technique. Although propofol anaesthesia allows earlier awakening, later recovery events, including the ultimate endpoint of hospital discharge, are not reached earlier with propofol compared to most volatile anaesthetics. It is possible that some of these comparisons were not made at equivalent depths of anaesthesia because of the use of "standardised" infusion regimens or fixed volatile anaesthetic concentrations.

Furthermore, the use of intravenous adjuvants such as fentanyl and midazolam may have masked small differences between techniques. Another possibility is that fixed recovery room and day case unit protocols may have prevented patients progressing to discharge as rapidly as the anaesthetic technique actually permitted. Nevertheless, it is equally likely that differences in recovery from propofol or volatile anaesthesia are of little clinical significance. However, the substitution of propofol for volatile anaesthetic agents appears to produce further improvements in the

85

incidence of PONV, even when propofol is used as an induction agent prior to an inhalational technique.

The use of propofol as a maintenance anaesthetic may also be advantageous for longer day case procedures, as emergence, recovery, and discharge times appear to be shorter after an extended propofol anaesthetic compared to isoflurane. This advantage of propofol may be less marked compared to the newer inhaled anaesthetics, however.

Use of opioids and other adjuvants

As propofol has no analgesic properties, it is often necessary to supplement its use with opioid analgesic drugs. Because opioid analgesics can also cause sedation and depression of mental function, short acting agents such as fentanyl and alfentanil are the most widely used analgesics in day case anaesthesia. They can often improve intraoperative conditions by reducing unwanted patient movements without significantly delaying recovery. An infusion of alfentanil may reduce the requirement for supplemental propofol boluses to treat clinical signs of inadequate anaesthesia.[3] Although opioid analgesics are a potent cause of PONV, the use of opioid supplements need not necessarily produce a substantial increase in this side effect.[3] Where the incidence of PONV is already high, however, the supplemental use of opioid analgesics may delay discharge due to the need to treat emetic sequelae.[4] In the future, the availability of the ultrashort acting opioid analgesic remifentanil may permit improved suppression of noxious stimuli when it is administered as an adjuvant during day case anaesthesia. It is hoped that the extremely short half time of this novel opioid will facilitate rapid recovery and limit the severity and duration of adverse postoperative side effects. However, the provision of effective analgesia in the postoperative period is likely to be problematic.

Because of the seriousness of PONV in the day case setting, there has been much interest in alternative analgesic agents. The NSAIDs are very useful for procedures associated with moderate levels of pain, but they cannot replace the opioid analgesics where more profound analgesia is required. Although the NSAIDs have a useful opioid sparing effect, this does not necessarily reduce the incidence or severity of PONV.[5] Nevertheless, the NSAIDs may produce longer lasting analgesia than commonly used opioids such as fentanyl. The α_2 agonists also have useful analgesic properties. A high incidence of CVS side effects, combined with residual sedation, may limit their utility in the day case setting, however. Short acting opioid analgesics can be used (with N_2O) as maintenance anaesthetics for day case surgery. The advantage of this technique appears to be faster awakening compared to volatile anaesthesia (although this can also be achieved with propofol). The use of opioid analgesics for anaesthetic maintenance has been associated with an unacceptably high incidence of intraoperative apnoea, PONV, and retching, however, while there is also a substantial risk of awareness. As a result, opioid analgesics are often used to supplement propofol but are rarely now used as the principal anaesthetic.

In summary, intravenous anaesthesia allows recovery which is at least as rapid and complete as that from inhalational agents following day case procedures. Although rapid recovery is highly relevant in the day case setting, absence of side effects, especially those which may delay or even prevent discharge, is equally important. Propofol has clinical properties that are particularly well suited to the field of day case anaesthesia. Specifically, it combines smooth, effective anaesthesia with rapid recovery and a favourable side effect profile. Propofol significantly reduces the incidence of PONV and has antiemetic properties. Although new iv anaesthetic agents continue to be developed, as yet there are none that can rival propofol in the day case setting. There is still a need for a potent analgesic devoid of the side effects of the opioids. Remifentanil is a step in the right direction, although its side effects are not prevented, merely limited in duration. At present, the use of a combination of low doses of several drugs appears the most beneficial in terms of reducing adverse effects.

Children

Total intravenous anaesthesia has taken rather longer to become popular in paediatric patients than in adults. This is in part due to children's inherent dislike of needles, which has tended to favour inhalation induction, logically followed by the use of an inhaled agent for maintenance. A second factor is the type of case encountered in paediatric anaesthesia, which is often of brief duration and until relatively recently would have resulted in delayed recovery had barbiturates rather than volatile anaesthetics been used. Finally, children do not have the acquired diseases of adults, with cardiovascular disease being especially uncommon (other than congenital cardiac defects). The relative cardiovascular stability associated with etomidate and the opioids was not really required in children.

The availability of EMLA cream and, more recently, topical amethocaine gel has made iv induction of anaesthesia more common in children. With the increased use of iv induction has also come more widespread use of iv drugs for maintenance of anaesthesia, especially since the availability of propofol and the newer opioids. This section will review the specialised applications of iv anaesthesia to children and also consider pharmacological differences from adults.

Hypnotic

Propofol

Propofol is the iv hypnotic most commonly used in children because its duration of action is most suited to the typical paediatric cases. Compared to adults, the volume of distribution of propofol in the central compartment is larger in children (340 ml/kg versus 230 ml/kg), and its clearance is greater (32–57 ml/kg/min versus 27 mg/kg/min). As a result, higher doses are required to achieve and maintain the same blood levels in children compared to adults. There may also be pharmacodynamic differences as the target concentration required to achieve and maintain adequate anaesthesia appears to be higher in children than in adults. Levels of 6·6 µg/ml may be required to prevent movement in response to surgical stimuli in children, compared to 5–6 µg/ml in adults. Pharmacokinetic studies in children should be interpreted with caution, however. Accurate data require frequent sampling of relatively large blood volumes, which may be impractical in small children, introducing errors. In practice, induction doses of 2·5–3·5 mg/kg followed by infusion rates of 100–300 µg/kg/min appear to be satisfactory in children.

True TIVA is very uncommon in paediatric practice; where propofol is used to maintain anaesthesia, it is almost always combined with N_2O as part of a balanced technique. Induction of anaesthesia with propofol in children results in reductions of 10–20% in heart rate and blood pressure, less than those observed in adults and generally within the clinically acceptable range. The relative absence of peripheral vascular disease in children makes hypotension somewhat more acceptable. Bradycardia may be more of a problem in children following the use of propofol, especially when it is administered with alfentanil or suxamethonium.

A common operation in children is strabismus surgery, which is associated with a high incidence of PONV. This undesirable side effect may occur in 60–80% of children when halothane is used as the main anaesthetic, but can be reduced to 16–20% by the use of propofol. Similar effects of propofol in reducing PONV have also been observed after other paediatric day case procedures. As in adults, eliminating N_2O and opioids may further reduce the incidence of PONV. The antiemetic effect of propofol, like its sedative effects, is shortlived, however, and emesis rates after discharge may be no different with propofol compared to alternative anaesthetics where the surgical procedure (e.g. strabismus repair) is the major cause of PONV.

Propofol may have some additional advantages in several specific groups of children. It is safe in malignant hyperpyrexia (MH) susceptible individuals and is widely used in patients at high risk for this complication. Propofol may be used during microlaryngoscopy when a tracheal tube cannot be used and where rapid emergence is required so that the patient can protect their airway. A catheter can be used for oxygen insufflation while anaesthesia is provided by a propofol infusion. N_2O can also be avoided, which is useful when the laser or cautery are being used as N_2O supports combustion. Propofol may also sufficiently attenuate upper airway reflexes to permit tracheal intubation without neuromuscular blocking drugs in patients with myasthenia gravis or other neuromuscular disorders. Propofol can also be used in this way as an alternative to suxamethonium, which is associated with more severe arrhythmias (and cardiac arrest) in normal children compared to adults. Subanaesthetic doses of propofol have also been used for sedation for radiological or diagnostic procedures, CT and MRI scans, radiotherapy, and cardiac catheterisation. Propofol infusions are also valuable in situations where anaesthetised patients have to be moved from one location to another.

Ketamine

Ketamine is also often used in children. It may be particularly useful in the uncontrollable child (as a last resort) as it can be given intramuscularly. Newer uses and routes of administration are also being found. Ketamine can be given orally or nasally for sedation prior to surgery and is also useful in a variety of repetitive, painful procedures including burns dressing changes or wound debridement. It is often used during cardiac catheterisation, as it has relatively little effect on cardiovascular and respiratory systems. Caution should still be exercised in the use of ketamine where operative decisions are to be made based on pulmonary vascular resistance, however, and as with other uses of ketamine, facilities and personnel to secure the airway may still be required.

Benzodiazepines

One of the major uses of benzodiazepines in children has been as an oral premedicant. The most effective drug seems to be midazolam and as no oral formulation is commercially available, the iv solution is used. Adding midazolam to a commercial analgesic (e.g. ibuprofen syrup) is useful, both to mask its bitter taste and also to provide a useful degree of postoperative pain relief. An oral dose of $0 \cdot 5–0 \cdot 75$ mg/kg is necessary because of the relatively low bioavailability. Intravenous midazolam has also been used as a sedative. As it has minimal effect on cardiac electrophysiology, it is useful during reentrant arrhythmia electrophysiological studies. Midazolam is also extensively used for sedation of children in the ICU.

The clearance of midazolam is somewhat slower in neonates than in older children, necessitating smaller doses to ensure rapid recovery. Pharmacokinetic data obtained from the paediatric population have been used to develop computer assisted continuous infusions of midazolam which have been used together with an opioid analgesic for cardiac surgery as an easily used alternative to volatile anaesthetics.

Opioids

The major use of opioid analgesics in the paediatric population is during cardiac surgery for the repair of congenital defects. Several years ago, it was demonstrated that deep intraoperative anaesthesia with a high dose opioid technique significantly reduced markers of the physiological stress response such as hyperglycaemia, lactic acidaemia, and elevated blood levels of acetoacetate compared to light anaesthesia with halothane and morphine.[6] In addition, the opioid based technique was associated with fewer serious outcomes, including sepsis, metabolic acidosis, disseminated intravascular coagulation, and death. The combination of opioids with a benzodiazepine can further improve haemodynamic stability and reduce the stress response during paediatric cardiac surgery. Opioids may also be used for sedation of children with congenital heart defects undergoing cardiac catheterisation. Interestingly, children with cyanotic heart disease appear to require a lower dose of opioids compared to those with non-cyanotic lesions.

Another area where opioid based iv anaesthetic techniques may be of benefit in children is during spinal surgery for scoliosis. The use of alfentanil with N_2O does not interfere with evoked cortical somatosensory potentials and also facilitates an intraoperative "wake-up" test should this be required, while still providing acceptable analgesia.[7]

The pharmacokinetics of opioids in children differ from those in adults in that the volume of distribution is approximately 50% greater and clearance is almost doubled. This suggests that children will require somewhat greater induction and maintenance doses (per kilogram) compared to adults. If the pharmacokinetic parameters are expressed with respect to body surface area rather than weight, however, the differences from adults are less apparent.

In summary, although iv anaesthesia has been less popular in children compared to adults, more recent drug developments have increased its use considerably. Children present different problems to adults and some of the procedures required in small children may be particularly well managed using iv techniques. For most drugs, children will require larger doses compared to adults but as always, careful observation and assessment of effect allow for the optimal titration of drugs.

The elderly

The elderly are an increasing element of the population and, because of their propensity to coexisting diseases, make up a substantial component of the anaesthetic population. The elderly are more sensitive to the CNS effects of intravenous anaesthetics, requiring reduced doses for a variety of reasons and being at increased risk for adverse effects. The impact of coexisting diseases may be of greater importance than chronological age and different systems are affected to varying degrees by age. Age related changes in pharmacokinetics include alterations in protein binding, body composition, tissue perfusion, and the function of excretory organs. Although plasma proteins change relatively little in the elderly, the presence of hepatic, renal or connective tissue diseases can induce much larger changes. With ageing there is a decrease in total body water and diminished lean body mass with an increase in fat content. This decreases the volume of distribution of water soluble drugs, but has the opposite effect for fat soluble drugs. Lean body mass is a better predictor of dose than weight in the elderly.

There is a decline in early diastolic left ventricular filling with ageing, decreasing tissue perfusion, thereby delaying the time to peak drug effect and reducing hepatic clearance. Reductions in liver mass and regional blood flow also reduce hepatic clearance with increasing age. Glomerular filtration and renal blood flow also decline with age, although a large amount of interpatient variability exists. These effects on renal and hepatic clearance may necessitate reduced doses and/or an increased dosing frequency (or lower infusion rates).

Alterations in pharmacodynamics with age involve reductions in the number and activity of CNS receptors. The affinity of receptors for neurotransmitter molecules is reduced within the CNS, while in the periphery, plasma levels of catecholamines are increased, although the end organs are less responsive. The interaction of these many factors on the actions of common iv anaesthetics will now be examined.

Hypnotics

The elderly require lower doses of barbiturates for induction of anaesthesia when compared with younger adults. This finding appears to be due to pharmacokinetic rather than pharmacodynamic effects. It has been demonstrated that the relationship between steady state plasma concentration and EEG effects of thiopentone are the same in young and elderly patients. The pharmacokinetics of thiopentone are heavily dependent upon body mass and cardiac function, both of which are altered in the elderly. These changes may explain most of the differences observed with thiopentone. The response of the elderly to an induction dose of thiopentone is more variable than in younger patients, requiring even greater care in drug administration.

The duration of barbiturates in the elderly is prolonged, through both altered redistribution and reduced metabolic clearance. The elderly are also more sensitive to etomidate, again for pharmacokinetic rather than pharmacodynamic reasons. Although the relative cardiovascular stability of etomidate may be desirable in the elderly, it may have significant negative inotropic effects in the presence of CVS disease.

The plasma concentration resulting from a given dose of propofol is somewhat greater in the elderly compared to younger adults. In addition, the pharmacodynamic effects of propofol appear to be exaggerated with ageing. As a result, the elderly are especially susceptible to hypotension following induction of anaesthesia with propofol. The total body clearance of propofol is also reduced in the elderly, resulting in delayed awakening.

Elderly patients with ischaemic heart disease may be more susceptible to the cardiostimulatory effects of ketamine. Ketamine induced hallucinations may also be more disorientating in an older population. Recovery from ketamine is not greatly altered in the elderly unless there is a significant reduction in hepatic blood flow or metabolic function.

Benzodiazepines

The elderly appear to be more sensitive to the central depressant effects of benzodiazepines. In contrast to the iv anaesthetics, this appears to be primarily a pharmacodynamic alteration rather than a difference in pharmacokinetics. It is likely that the enhanced sensitivity is due to changes in benzodiazepine receptor occupancy, although no age related differences in receptor number or affinity have been demonstrated. Reduced clearance of benzodiazepines occurs in the elderly with prolongation of their actions, especially in the presence of hepatic dysfunction. As in younger patients, midazolam allows the fastest recovery. The other benzodiazepines may be especially prolonged in the presence of liver disease as they have active metabolites.

Opioids

Elderly patients demonstrate increased sensitivity to all the opioid analgesics. This is a result of both pharmacokinetic and pharmacodynamic differences. Opioid induced ventilatory depression occurs frequently in the elderly and may be more profound and of longer duration compared to younger patients.

Remifentanil, the new esterase metabolised opioid, has not yet been extensively evaluated in the elderly. Preliminary evidence suggests that older patients are just as susceptible to the hypotensive and ventilatory depressant effects of this drug as they are to the other opioids. The non-specific esterase metabolism of remifentanil does not appear to be reduced with age, however, and remifentanil appears to be just as short acting in old patients as it is in younger ones. This brief duration of action of remifentanil will limit the duration of those adverse effects which do occur in the elderly.

Muscle relaxants and their antagonists

Most of the muscle relaxants have a prolonged duration of action in the elderly, especially in the presence of severe renal or hepatic dysfunction. Suxamethonium is an exception. Although levels of pseudocholinesterase decrease with ageing, this has a clinically negligible effect on suxamethonium's duration of action. Atracurium and cis-atracurium, which can be eliminated by Hofmann degradation, are also not markedly prolonged, although their duration may be extended by an altered volume of distribution. The onset of rocuronium, usually comparable to that of suxamethonium, may be delayed due to decreased cardiac output. As with younger patients, considerable interpatient variability exists in the response to neuromuscular blocking drugs. As excellent monitors of neuromuscular block are readily available and easy to interpret, they should be used routinely to guide dosage and especially redosing.

Because most muscle relaxants are prolonged in the elderly, reversal agents are more likely to be required. The duration of neostigmine is prolonged, although that of edrophonium is considerably shortened and a larger dose is required for a comparable effect in the elderly. The combined effects of anticholinergic and anticholinesterase drugs should, in theory, not alter heart rate or rhythm. In practice, dysrrhythmias are often observed, although these are less common after glycopyrrolate compared to atropine. Glycopyrrolate is a more logical choice than atropine in elderly patients for this reason, but also because its duration of effect is more closely matched to that of neostigmine. Finally, as glycopyrrolate does not enter the CNS, it does not produce the confusion sometimes observed in elderly patients from the central anticholinergic syndrome.

In summary, ageing has a variable and unpredictable effect on the actions and durations of a number of iv drugs. These changes are often the result of, or exacerbated by, deterioration of essential organ function. Intravenous drugs still have advantages over inhaled anaesthetics in elderly patients but they must be administered cautiously, using small doses and with careful monitoring of the resultant effects.

Critically ill patients

Anaesthesia for critically ill patients is complicated because of an interplay of multiple factors. Important issues which must be addressed are the effects of anaesthetics on critical organ systems which may already be severely compromised, how changes in physiology affect distribution of and responses to anaesthetic drugs and how alterations in hepatic and renal function affect drug elimination and hence duration of effect. The critical system most affected by, and having the greatest effect on, iv anaesthetics is the cardiovascular system (CVS). A number of CVS problems in the critically ill will now be reviewed.

Hypovolaemia is common in critically ill patients. In the presence of hypovolaemia, compensatory responses occur, including central catecholamine release and sympathetic stimulation, which help to maintain the systemic blood pressure by way of tachycardia and vasoconstriction. In addition to their direct effects on myocardial contractility and peripheral vascular resistance, iv anaesthetics also inhibit central catecholamine output and the baroreceptor reflex, which tends to overcome the effects of these compensatory mechanisms. As a result, the depressant effects of the iv anaesthetics on blood pressure may be considerably magnified.

The haemodynamic effects of various iv anaesthetics differ, with propofol being the most depressant, thiopentone and midazolam intermediate, and etomidate the least depressant. Even etomidate may cause a marked reduction in blood pressure in the presence of severe hypovolaemia, however. Despite this, the effect of iv anaesthetics on the baroreceptor reflex is less than that observed with some volatile anaesthetics. Clearly, intravascular volume should be restored as much as possible prior to induction of anaesthesia. Ketamine is unusual amongst the iv induction agents because it can increase the heart rate, blood pressure, and cardiac output in critically ill patients.[8] This occurs because ketamine blocks the reuptake of monoamines (e.g. noradrenaline) into adrenergic nerves, resulting in an increase in sympathetic activity. When there has been prolonged sympathetic stimulation, however, there may be depletion of catecholamines, preventing the sympathomimetic effects of ketamine and unmasking its direct negative inotropic and vasodilator effects. Consequently, ketamine can result in cardiovascular depression in some critically ill patients.

An alternative strategy to minimise CVS depression is the high dose opioid technique. The use of opioids alone may be associated with prolonged ventilatory depression and delayed recovery, however, and the technique also introduces a greater risk of intraoperative awareness. There is a tendency, therefore, to use combinations of iv drugs in order to minimise the adverse effects of each component, while providing the optimal effect from the drug combination. Unlike volatile anaesthetics, once an iv drug has been administered, it cannot be removed other than via redistribution and elimination. Great care is therefore required in order to prevent overdosage, giving a small initial dose and not administering additional drug until adequate time has been allowed for it to achieve its maximum effect. Drugs which rapidly equilibrate with their effect site are much easier to use in this situation as peak effect will be achieved sooner. The altered cardiovascular state and redistribution of blood flow may alter the time to peak effect of some drugs, however.

While avoiding hypotension on induction of anaesthesia, it is also important to prevent or minimise the hypertensive response to tracheal intubation. Opioids are commonly administered with iv anaesthetics for this purpose. Unfortunately, concomitant delivery of opioid analgesics can enhance the decrease in blood pressure following induction of anaesthesia. It is also important to consider the timing of drug delivery, so that tracheal intubation occurs at the time of peak effect of both iv hypnotic and analgesic. Optimum effects appear to result from a moderate dose of opioid and a small dose of hypnotic, rather than a high iv anaesthetic dose with less opioid. Alfentanil is a good choice of opioid in the critically ill as it has a short time to peak effect and also allows a more rapid recovery from its respiratory depressant properties.

Although propofol is associated with hypotension on induction of anaesthesia, when ventricular function is impaired, the elevated cardiac filling pressures may benefit from vasodilation secondary to propofol. Propofol is also more likely to permit early extubation because of its favourable recovery profile.

Control of heart rate is also important in critically ill patients. Bradycardia is undesirable if it decreases cardiac output. Tachycardia is also undesirable as it reduces the time for coronary perfusion and adversely affects the myocardial oxygen supply and demand ratio. Bradycardia is likely with the use of high dose opioid techniques, especially in the presence of β blockers and calcium antagonists. Concomitant use of pancuronium (or rocuronium) as the muscle relaxant may be beneficial as their vagolytic properties will counter the vagal effect of opioids without producing significant tachycardia. In the presence of severe bradycardia, cholinergic medications may be required. The unpredictable response to these drugs may result in a rebound tachycardia, however. An alternative approach may be the use of an oesophageal atrial pacing electrode which can treat bradycardia faster than either atropine or glycopyrrolate and allows any chosen heart rate to be maintained.[9]

Care should also be exercised in the use of reversal drugs to antagonise residual neuromuscular block as these drugs also have an unpredictable effect on heart rate. Allowing neuromuscular block to recover spontaneously, even if a period of postoperative respiratory support is required, may be the safest option.

For severely haemodynamically unstable patients, little (if any) iv anaesthesia should be used. Instead, an opioid analgesic, supplemented with a small dose of benzodiazepine, can produce an unconscious amnesic state. The use of the benzodiazepine is important, as critically ill patients have subsequently had recall when they were given minimal anaesthesia because of extreme hypotension or even circulatory arrest. If the condition of the patient improves, additional benzodiazepine or a low dose of an iv anaesthetic can be added. It should be recalled that combinations of benzodiazepines and opioids are synergistic for both hypnotic and respiratory depressant effects.

It is also important to preserve cerebral perfusion pressure in critically ill patients. This can be achieved by avoiding decreases in systemic blood pressure and increases in intracranial pressure.

In contrast to the volatile anaesthetics, intravenous agents cause cerebral vasoconstriction and metabolic depression.[10] In addition, the volatile anaesthetics also impair cerebral autoregulation and uncouple blood flow from metabolism. With the exception of ketamine, which causes hypertension and increases intracranial pressure, all iv anaesthetics cause cerebrovascular constriction and reduction in $CMRO_2$. The cardiovascular depressant effects of these iv agents may reduce cerebral perfusion pressure, however, especially if there is preexisting CVS compromise. In the presence of CVS disease, the use of opioid analgesics with a reduced dose of hypnotic will minimise hypotension, while attenuating the increase in blood pressure (and intracranial pressure) accompanying tracheal intubation. Provided its hypotensive effects can be attenuated, propofol is ideal in head injuries because of its beneficial effects on cerebral perfusion combined with rapid recovery.

The effects of altered physiology on pharmacokinetics should also be taken into account. Major illnesses alter tissue blood flow, fluid compartment volumes, plasma protein levels, and end organ metabolic function. These changes may alter drug kinetics. In addition, the concomitant use of inotropes or vasodilators may also alter the behaviour of anaesthetic drugs. Ischaemia may lead to metabolic acidosis, altering the ionisation of drugs and their degree of plasma protein binding. Redistribution of a reduced cardiac output to critical areas (e.g. CNS) may result in a higher proportion of an induction dose reaching the brain, with an exacerbation of central depressant effects.

Impaired hepatic blood flow or liver function may delay recovery from the sedative effects of drugs such as midazolam and propofol. Muscle relaxants like vecuronium may also have a prolonged effect in the presence of hepatic or renal dysfunction. Because atracurium and cis-atracurium are eliminated by Hofmann degradation, they are the agents of choice in organ dysfunction. Of the two, cis-atracurium causes less histamine release and less CVS depression.

For rapid sequence intubation, suxamethonium may be used although hyperkalaemia following burns and denervation injuries, as well as a host of other side effects, may complicate its use. Rocuronium is a viable alternative to suxamethonium in terms of onset, although, like vecuronium, it may be prolonged by hepatorenal dysfunction.

In summary, because of the interplay of a variety of factors, including altered perfusion, changed protein binding, abnormal volumes of distribution and clearances, and altered sensitivity to sedative drugs, it is difficult to predict the exact behaviour of a given drug in a particular patient. Critically ill patients show greater than usual variability in their responses to anaesthetics and analgesics. The cautious use of small doses of appropriately chosen drugs in proven combinations, with careful assessment of drug effect and modification of dosing intervals where necessary, will result in the best patient outcome.

Summary

All the above four special groups will encompass a wide range of patient types and surgical procedures, necessitating individual anaesthetic regimens. Nevertheless, it may be helpful to indicate some typical anaesthetic regimens and commonly used doses, with the proviso that these may require considerable modification in many cases.

For adult day cases, typical induction doses would be midazolam 1–3 mg followed by propofol 1·5–2·5 mg/kg. For maintenance, a variable rate propofol infusion of 75–200 µg/kg/min is usually required, supplemented by an infusion of alfentanil 0·5–1 µg/kg/min or perhaps now remifentanil 0·1–0·2 µg/kg/min. Children are ideally premedicated with oral midazolam 0·5–0·75 mg/kg followed by iv propofol 2·5–3·5 mg/kg and an infusion of 100–300 µg/kg/min, supplemented by N_2O. Elderly patients may receive midazolam 1–2 mg (primarily to minimise the hypotensive effects of propofol) followed by propofol 0·5–1·5 mg/kg or etomidate 0·1–0·2 mg/kg. A propofol infusion rate of 50–100 µg/kg/min is likely to be sufficient, supplemented, if necessary, by alfentanil 0·25–0·75 µg/kg/min or remifentanil 0·05–0·15 µg/kg/min. Drug doses based on lean (rather than actual) body weight are less likely to produce adverse effects. In critically ill patients, adequate resuscitation should precede anaesthetic induction whenever possible. Anaesthetic induction should comprise midazolam 1–2 mg and alfentanil 10–20 µg/kg (for amnesia and haemodynamic stability), supplemented (if cardiovascular status permits) by etomidate 0·1–0·2 mg/kg or ketamine 1–2 mg/kg. The maintenance analgesic and anaesthetic are best titrated to clinical response and the condition of the patient.

It must be stressed that the dose ranges for all these patient groups are only suggestions and must be adapted to suit individual circumstances.

1 Smith I, White PF, Nathanson M, Gouldson R. Propofol: an update on its clinical use. *Anesthesiology* 1994;**81**:1005–43.
2 Borgeat A, Wilder-Smith OHG, Suter PM. The nonhypnotic therapeutic applications of propofol. *Anesthesiology* 1994;**80**:642–56.
3 Smith I, Van Hemelrijck J, White PF. Efficacy of esmolol versus alfentanil as a supplement to propofol-N_2O anesthesia. *Anesth Analg* 1991;**73**:540–6.
4 Sukhani R, Vazquez J, Pappas AL, *et al*. Recovery after propofol with and without intraoperative fentanyl in patients undergoing ambulatory gynecologic laparoscopy. *Anesth Analg* 1996;**83**:975–81.
5 Smith I, White PF. New anaesthetics, analgesics and muscle relaxants for ambulatory surgery. *Curr Opin Anaesthesiol* 1995;**8**:298–303.
6 Anand KJ, Hickey PR. Halothane-morphine compared with high-dose sufentanil for anesthesia and postoperative analgesia in neonatal cardiac surgery. *NEJM* 1992;**362**:1–9.
7 Van Beem H, van Koopman GA, Kruls H, Notermans SL. Spinal monitoring during vertebral column surgery under continuous alfentanil infusion. *Eur J Anaesthesiol* 1992;**9**:287–91.
8 Lippman M, Appel PL, Mok MS, Shoemaker WC. Sequential cardiorespiratory patterns of anesthesia induction with ketamine in critically ill patients. *Crit Care Med* 1983;**11**:730–4.
9 Smith I, Monk TG, White PF. Comparison of transesophageal atrial pacing with anticholinergic drugs for the treatment of intraoperative bradycardia. *Anesth Analg* 1994;**78**:245–52.
10 Ravussin P, de Tribolet N, Wilder-Smith OHG. Total intravenous anesthesia is best for neurologic surgery. *J Neurosurg Anesth* 1994;**6**:285–9.

5: Intravenous anaesthesia delivery and monitoring systems

Introduction

Inhalation anaesthesia requires a delivery system, the calibrated vaporiser. Although these devices are quite complex and it is usually necessary to make several adjustments to the dial setting during the course of an anaesthetic, inhalation anaesthesia is perceived as relatively simple, a reflection of our familiarity with its use. Intravenous anaesthesia also requires a dedicated delivery system and periodic adjustments of drug delivery in order to produce a satisfactory anaesthetic state. This chapter will examine the various delivery systems which are available, from the simple to the complex, and describe their optimum use during anaesthesia. If drug delivery is to be adjusted or titrated, it is essential to know against which endpoint(s) this adjustment needs to be made. We will therefore examine the various parameters which can be monitored during anaesthesia and describe their usefulness in regulating intravenous anaesthesia. In addition to the routinely measured effects of anaesthesia and surgery, stress hormones are frequently secreted during and after surgical procedures. We will review this stress response and discuss the various strategies which have been employed for its control and examine their effect on subsequent outcome.

Intravenous drug delivery systems

The basic equipment needed to deliver iv anaesthetics, a syringe and hollow needle, was developed in the mid 18th century. For induction of anaesthesia, it is still common to manually administer a bolus dose, observing the effect and stopping drug delivery when the desired endpoint (e.g. loss of consciousness) is achieved. Because it takes time for the drug to diffuse from the circulation into the site of its effect, a relative overdose is likely to be administered (from the drug yet to reach the effect site when delivery ceases), potentially producing adverse effects such as hypotension.

This problem can be reduced somewhat by slower drug administration, allowing more time for equilibration between plasma and effect site, as well as by using drugs which reach the effect site more rapidly (e.g. alfentanil rather than fentanyl). As the effect of the initial (induction) dose wears off through redistribution, it will be necessary to deliver more drug if it is desired to maintain the effect (i.e. to maintain anaesthesia). This can be achieved in a number of ways, each of which has advantages and disadvantages (table 5.1). The simplest method is to inject further boluses of drug, although this approach tends to result in plasma concentrations which oscillate from peaks of relatively excessive drug concentrations to troughs of inadequate amount (fig 5.1).

These peaks may be associated with adverse effects such as hypotension and apnoea, the latter being problematic if it is intended to maintain spontaneous ventilation, while the troughs may result in inadequate anaesthesia. A more stable anaesthetic can be achieved by using a continuous infusion in order to maintain relatively constant drug levels without fluctuating from inadequate to excessive anaesthesia (fig 5.2). Compared to intermittent bolus administration, a continuous infusion smoothes out the peaks and troughs (reducing side effects), but also results in a reduced total amount of anaesthetic being delivered so that recovery may actually occur earlier.[1] The delivery of continuous infusions requires more equipment than bolus dosing. Although relatively simple flow regulators can be used, this type of apparatus is relatively crude and offers

Table 5.1   Advantages and disadvantages of alternative methods for iv drug delivery

Technique	Advantages	Disadvantages
Intermittent boluses	Simple No special equipment required	Poor quality of anaesthesia (peaks and troughs) Large total drug dose Slow recovery
Fixed rate infusion	Possibly smoother anaesthesia	Anaesthesia "deepens" with time Risk of awareness or side effects (depending upon chosen rate)

Variable infusion	Smoother anaesthesia
	Lower total drug dose
	Faster recovery
	  (versus intermittent bolus)
		Frequent adjustments needed
		May be difficult to titrate
		  (lack of suitable clinical endpoints)

Stepped infusion	Achieves approximately stable
	  plasma concentration
	Computer not required
		Inflexible
		Difficult to superimpose changes in
		  response to clinical effect

Target controlled infusion	Achieves approximately stable
	  plasma concentration
	Easy to superimpose changes in
	  response to clinical effect
		Considerable interpatient variability
		Expensive
		Further evaluation desirable

Closed loop infusion	Eliminates pharmacokinetic and pharmacodynamic variability	Lack of suitable endpoints Not yet practical for anaesthetics

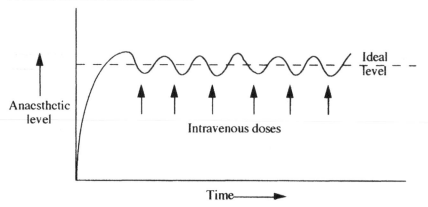

Fig 5.1   Level of anaesthesia resulting from a loading bolus dose of intravenous drug followed by repeated injection of further small boluses. The ideal (or target) level of anaesthesia is indicated by a dotted line

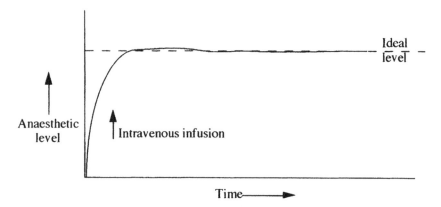

Fig 5.2   Level of anaesthesia resulting from a loading bolus dose of intravenous drug followed by a continuous infusion. The ideal (or target) level of anaesthesia is indicated by a dotted line

little control over the rate of administration of potent drugs. Although such equipment is more reliable with dilute drug solutions, this may result in a considerable fluid load.

Infusion pumps designed for use in the ICU can also be used to deliver iv anaesthetic drugs. These devices are usually syringe drivers (fig 5.3) designed to provide relatively constant rates of drug delivery. When used for iv anaesthesia, however, these pumps may not be sufficiently flexible. For example, it is often desirable to deliver both induction and maintenance doses from the same system. This will necessitate a relatively rapid rate of delivery (e.g. 1000 ml/h) for induction, as well as much slower rates (e.g.

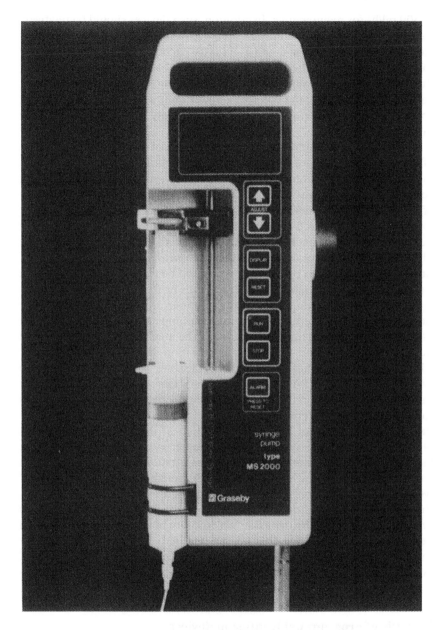

Fig 5.3   A simple syringe driver infusion pump. The device is calibrated to deliver a specified volume every hour, which is set using the up and down arrow keys. Changes in infusion rates can only be made with the pump stopped

0–300 ml/h) for maintenance. In addition, such devices should be relatively robust, being resistant to fluids, interference from radiofrequency and other electromagnetic fields, and other hazards encountered in the operating theatre environment. The pump should be capable of being operated from the mains electricity supply, but with a rechargeable battery to allow continued operation in the event of a power failure or in remote locations, as well as to provide a back-up power supply to retain programme information.

An ideal infusion pump should also be capable of operating with a variety of different sized syringes (even from different manufacturers). Many of the modern pumps automatically sense the size of syringe in use, requesting conformation by the user prior to drug delivery. This facility will reduce errors from the pump delivering an inappropriate rate of plunger movement for the syringe in use and thereby infusing drug at an incorrect rate. Syringe pumps should also incorporate a mechanism to ensure that the syringe plunger is correctly located and retained to prevent passive siphoning of drug into patients. This phenomenon can also be reduced by never placing a syringe pump at a height above the patient's heart.

Most iv drugs are administered as a dose per unit weight or weight and time. In contrast, however, simple infusion pumps are calibrated in volume of drug delivered over time. This requires the anaesthetist to calculate the pump settings based on the drug concentration and the patient's weight. More sophisticated pumps allow these variables to be entered into the syringe driver, along with the desired delivery rate which is entered directly in mg/kg/h or µg/kg/min (fig 5.4). An inbuilt microprocessor then performs the necessary calculations and sets the actual infusion rate. Most infusion devices use a numerical keypad for the input of this type of information, although an alternative system (Infus[OR], Baxter Healthcare) uses magnetic "smart" labels to programme the drug concentration and simple dials to set patient weight and flow rates (fig 5.5). Although these dials only allow weight and infusion rates to be entered in discrete steps (e.g. 55, 60, 70 kg), this lack of precision is not especially important in routine practice and is offset to some degree by the easier accessibility of the dials compared to a keypad when infusion rate changes are required. Inadvertent rate adjustments can be made just as easily as deliberate changes with such a system, however. Other devices use "menus" to select particular drugs, automatically setting an appropriate drug concentration for the chosen agent.

Hazards of programmable infusion devices

Although infusion pumps with inbuilt calculators prevent errors from incorrect calculation of flow rates, they may introduce other hazards. For example, some pumps can operate in a variety of "modes", such as mg/kg/h, µg/kg/min, and ml/h. It is possible to enter a numerical value

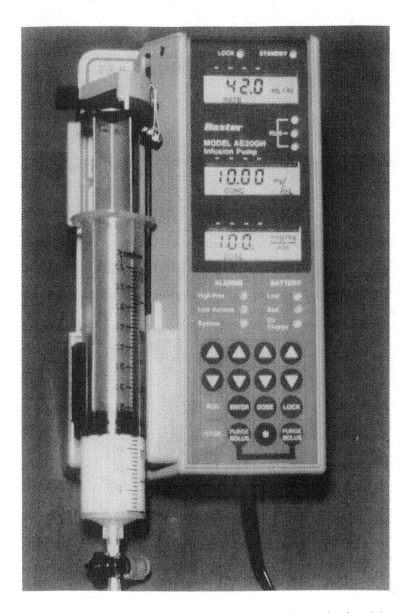

Fig 5.4 A programmable syringe driver infusion pump. The patient's weight and the drug concentration are entered using the numerical keys and the device then delivers a specified dose per kilogram per minute

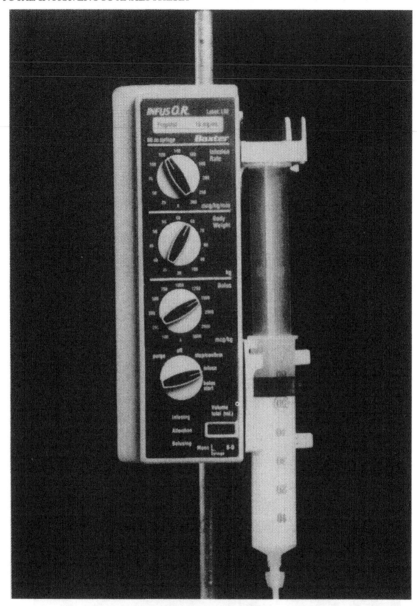

Fig 5.5 A programmable pump with interchangeable magnetic (smart) labels which convey information on drug concentration and appropriate bolus and infusion rates. The upper three dials set the infusion rate, patient's weight, and bolus dose, respectively, while the lower dial turns the pump on and off and initiates bolus delivery. Dose adjustments are easy with the simple dials and can be made with the pump running

which is correct for one mode of delivery but totally inappropriate if the pump happens to be in an alternative mode. Entering a desired rate of 160 μg/kg/h ($\approx$ 10 mg/kg/h) as "160" when the infusion pump is actually in a mg/kg/h mode will result in an almost 17-fold overdose. Such errors are not uncommon when one display screen is used for large amounts of information. Interestingly, very similar problems have occurred in the airline industry, with at least one modern aircraft crash being attributed to the pilot entering an excessively steep angle of approach when it was believed that an appropriate rate of descent was being input. Such disasters can be avoided by ensuring that only one type of information is entered in any given display field or by making the display of information clearly very different in each mode. Adequate training and raising practitioners' awareness of the possibility of such problems are also beneficial.

Infusion regimens

Once the equipment is available for iv drug delivery, the practitioner has to know what infusion rate to set for a desired effect and how this infusion rate must be adjusted in order to maintain that effect. For drugs which fit a three compartment model (e.g. propofol and the potent opioids), a bolus followed by a constant infusion will not result in a constant effect site concentration (see chapter 1). The initial infusion rate will need to be high to compensate for rapid drug redistribution, but will subsequently need to be reduced as the rate of redistribution slows and a steady state is approached. It would be relatively easy to adjust the infusion rate if it were possible to monitor the plasma drug concentration in the same way that end expired anaesthetic concentration is continuously displayed. All that would be required to achieve the desired level would be simple increases or decreases in the infusion rate. Unfortunately, real time measurement of the plasma concentration of intravenous anaesthetic drugs is not possible. Nevertheless, it is possible to take blood samples (preferably arterial) at known intervals after a drug bolus or short infusion and to measure the plasma drug concentrations in the laboratory using gas chromatography. In this way, it is possible to know with hindsight what the plasma concentration was at various times after particular dosing regimens. This information can then be incorporated into pharmacokinetic equations in order to determine the rate constants governing the movement of drugs between compartments (chapter 1). In turn, these constants can be used in a mathematical model in order to generate an infusion regimen which should maintain a particular blood concentration of a given anaesthetic drug. Naturally, as these values are obtained from a relatively small number of subjects, applying the resulting models to other individuals is associated with all the usual statistical variability associated with extrapolating from samples to larger populations.

Manual infusions

Using pharmacokinetic principles, it is possible to design an infusion regimen based upon a bolus dose followed by a manually adjusted stepped infusion. By making a few relatively minor simplifications, the steps can be reduced to only one or two rate changes over time. Making these steps manually has the advantage that any existing infusion system can be used (table 5.1). Such a regimen has been described for the delivery of propofol anaesthesia.[2] This regimen is designed to achieve and maintain a fixed blood concentration of propofol (3 μg/ml) and consists of a bolus of 1 mg/kg, followed by an infusion of 10 mg/kg/h for ten minutes, reduced to 8 mg/kg/h for ten minutes and culminating in an infusion of 6 mg/kg/h for the remainder of the anaesthetic. Although such a scheme achieves an approximation to constant plasma levels, it still lacks flexibility and may require supplementation with other anaesthetic or analgesic agents. Using the 10:8:6 propofol infusion regimen with 70% N_2O (and opioid premedication), it was still necessary to use a supplemental volatile anaesthetic in 25% of spontaneously breathing patients undergoing body surface surgery.[3] Further disadvantages of manually adjusted infusion regimens include the need to alter the infusion rate at set intervals, with the possibility of overdose if the anaesthetist is distracted from this task by other aspects of patient care. In addition, these schemes are designed to produce constant (fixed) plasma levels. Variations in the level of surgical stimulation or in patient susceptibility to a given concentration of anaesthetic drug may alter the anaesthetic requirements as there is no single blood concentration which will produce satisfactory anaesthesia at all levels of stimulation in all patients. The manual infusion schemes are too inflexible to allow changes in desired plasma concentration to be readily superimposed on the basic infusion regimen. Titration of iv anaesthetics is made more difficult by the need for the drug to diffuse to its effect site in order to produce a clinical response.

Computer control

Although the kinetics of drug distribution and diffusion into the effect site can be calculated, predicting the effect site concentration at any point during drug administration is complex. These problems can be overcome by incorporating all the necessary pharmacokinetic parameters (obtained from an appropriate patient population) into a computer which is allowed to automatically adjust the rate of drug delivery (fig 5.6). Because drug is delivered to achieve a desired (or target) concentration, these systems are known as target controlled infusion (TCI) systems. The acronym CACI (computer assisted continuous infusion) has also been used in the past.

TCI systems have been developed for propofol and alfentanil. A variety of investigative groups have been developing different TCI systems for some time. In late 1996, the first commercially available TCI system for the delivery of propofol (Diprifusor™) was launched (fig 5.7), based on the developmental work of Professor Gavin Kenny from Glasgow. Using a TCI system requires the anaesthetist to enter the patient's weight as well as their age, as pharmacokinetic parameters vary with age. An initial "target" blood propofol concentration is entered, following which the software instructs the pump to deliver a rapid infusion calculated to achieve this target concentration (fig 5.8). Subsequently, the computer continues to administer an infusion, the rate of which is constantly adjusted in order to maintain the set target concentration. If the resulting level of anaesthesia is clinically inappropriate, a new target concentration can be entered at any time. If this new target is higher than the current concentration, the system will deliver a further rapid infusion in order to attain the revised target. If a lower concentration is chosen, the software will stop drug infusion until it calculates that the plasma concentration has declined to the new target concentration, after which the infusion will be restarted at a rate sufficient to maintain the new target level. The use of a TCI system to deliver a constant plasma concentration which is then compared with clinical response is similar in concept to the use of a calibrated vaporiser to deliver a constant inspired anaesthetic concentration which is titrated against effect. In comparison to manually adjusted regimens, TCI propofol has

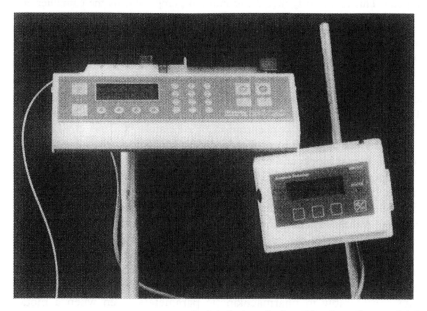

Fig 5.6 A prototype target controlled infusion device. The box (lower right) contains the computer and pharmacokinetic data and allows the patient's age and weight to be entered using a thumb wheel (on the left of the box). The computer sends instructions via a cable to a conventional syringe driver infusion pump (upper left)

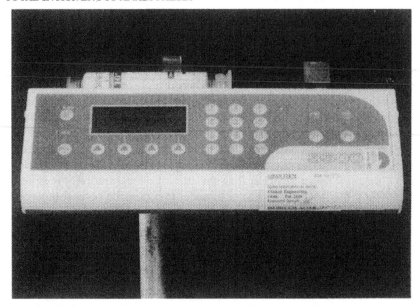

Fig 5.7 The Diprifusor™ commercial target controlled infusion pump for propofol. This modified syringe driver infusion pump contains the computer and pharmacokinetic data for propofol. The special prefilled propofol cartridge incorporates a magnetic label which confirms the presence of 1% propofol and enables the target controlled delivery mode. The device functions as a simple syringe driver infusion pump if conventional syringes are loaded in place of the propofol cartridge

been shown to be superior with respect to cardiovascular stability and ease of use during anaesthesia.[4] TCI systems can also be used for sedation by selecting a lower target concentration of propofol. TCI has already been used to deliver propofol to provide sedation for endoscopy, surgery under local or regional block, and on the ICU.

The performance of a TCI system can be evaluated by taking blood samples for laboratory measurement of actual measured blood concentrations of anaesthetic drug and retrospectively comparing these with the predicted values. Factors influencing the performance of these systems include the ability of the infusion pump to deliver drug at the precise rate dictated by the software, errors in the pharmacokinetic model (due to inappropriate methodology and data collection) and interpatient variability. The latter factor is probably the most important as an individual may differ quite considerably in pharmacokinetic parameters, even when a model based on a closely matched population is chosen.

Figure 5.9 illustrates the differences between actual measured and predicted propofol concentrations for a variety of pharmacokinetic models. It is clearly important that the pharmacokinetic model is appropriate for the

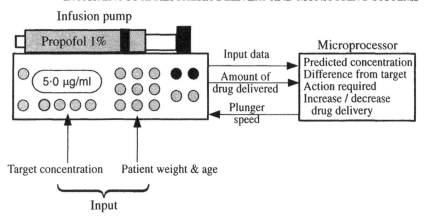

Fig 5.8 Diagram showing the principles of the target controlled infusion system. The user enters the patient's age, weight, and target concentration using the numeric keys. The microprocessor (contained within the syringe pump) calculates the predicted plasma concentration at any time, computes the difference between predicted and target concentration, determines whether more or less drug delivery is required, and sets an appropriate speed of syringe plunger movement to achieve the desired rate of infusion. The actual movement of the plunger is measured and constantly compared with the instructed rate of movement

specific patient population in which it is to be applied. For example, use of data derived from children resulted in improved performance of a TCI system in a paediatric population than when adult values were used.

A further source of error is pharmacodynamic variability. Even if it were possible to measure actual plasma iv drug concentrations in real time, there is a large variability between individuals in the level required to prevent a response to a given stimulus.[6] For these reasons, it is likely that TCI will be used in a similar way to a calibrated vaporiser. In other words, the anaesthetist will use the computer to deliver a relatively constant plasma concentration which will be adjusted in response to clinical signs, rather than relying on a specific target concentration at all times and for all patients. It is important, therefore, to determine how TCI systems perform compared to alternative forms of drug delivery (table 5.1).

Using a target controlled infusion of propofol designed to achieve a propofol concentration of 5 μg/ml, anaesthesia was induced successfully within three minutes in 90% of patients premedicated with temazepam.[4] TCI also reduced the magnitude of the reduction in MAP and the incidence of apnoea and pain on injection compared to manual bolus delivery. This more "gentle" induction of anaesthesia was achieved at the expense of a substantially longer time to loss of consciousness, however.

Fentanyl and alfentanil have also been delivered by TCI and are reported to improve haemodynamic stability compared to manual delivery. TCI

109

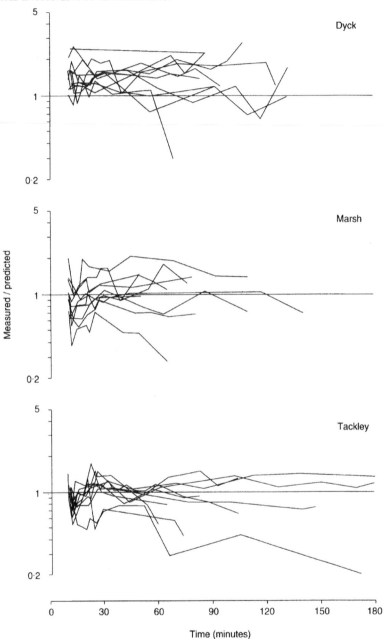

Fig 5.9 Ratio of measured to predicted arterial propofol concentration over time for each patient when propofol was delivered by one of three pharmacokinetic models. Values are plotted on a semilogarithmic scale. Reproduced with permission[5]

Table 5.2 Comparison of target controlled infusion (TCI) of propofol with propofol-halothane in children. Data from[7]

	Propofol-halothane	TCI propofol
Number (n)	20	20
Age (months)	67·6	66
	(16–154)	(13–141)
Duration (min)	30·6	33·3
	(9–52)	(11–60)
Adequate anaesthesia (%)	100	100
Emergence (min)	10·5	13·5
	(3–32)	(4–36)

Values are mean (range) or numbers (n)

systems appear to be relatively easy to learn to use and improve confidence in anaesthetists with little previous experience with TIVA. Although TCI systems are described as analogous to a vaporiser, only one study has so far compared TCI propofol to an inhaled anaesthetic.[7] In this randomised evaluation, comparable recovery times were achieved in children using either technique (table 5.2), although the volatile anaesthetic chosen was halothane, usually associated with delayed recovery. Further comparisons of TCI with alternative techniques are required before the final place of this technique is known.

Comparisons between volatile and iv anaesthetics are made difficult by uncertainty as to what constitutes an equipotent dose of the different anaesthetics. The potency of volatile agents is usually quoted in terms of the minimum alveolar concentration (MAC) of the anaesthetic required to prevent purposeful movement in 50% of patients in response to a skin incision. The effective blood concentration (EC_{50}) of propofol required to prevent response to surgical incision in 50% of patients has also been determined.[8] A value of 6·0 μg/ml prevented movement in half the patients when propofol was used alone, while a concentration of 6·2 μg/ml prevented movement in 95% of subjects (EC_{95}). Just as N_2O reduces the MAC of volatile anaesthetics, the presence of 67% N_2O reduced the EC_{50} of propofol to 4·5 μg/ml and the EC_{95} to 4·7 μg/ml.[8]

Closed loop systems

The process of drug delivery could be automated via a feedback loop if there was a reliable endpoint against which to monitor drug effect (fig 5.10). For providing analgesia, the patient's satisfaction with their pain relief can be used as such an endpoint and the wide variety of patient controlled analgesia (PCA) systems in current use represent a type of closed loop system. Similar systems have been modified to allow patients to administer hypnotic agents to provide conscious sedation. These patient controlled sedation (PCS) devices have generally proved popular with

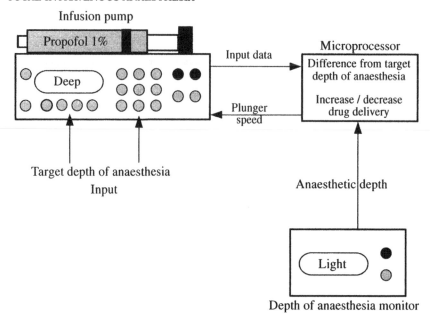

Fig 5.10 Simple feedback loop involving depth of anaesthesia monitor and target anaesthetic depth. The microprocessor simply requests more or less drug delivery in order to match the actual anaesthetic level to the desired value

patients and compare well with traditional techniques. Recently, a system has been described in which patients interact with a TCI infusion system to alter the target concentration of propofol in order to produce a more constant effect than conventional PCS. Patients can use a simple button to request a higher propofol concentration, whereas in the absence of regular patient requests, the plasma propofol concentration is permitted to decline gradually.[9] In this way, a patient who is oversedated (and therefore unable to continue to press their request button) will gradually awaken from sedation.

In order to deliver true closed loop control during anaesthesia, it will be necessary to have a reliable measurement of the "depth" of anaesthesia. Many systems have been evaluated as possible depth of anaesthesia monitors (see below), most of which are based on some form of processed EEG. A few prototype closed loop systems, based on either the EEG or auditory evoked potentials, have been used with moderate success, although these systems remain highly experimental and are unlikely to see widespread use in the near future. It is possible to monitor the endpoint of muscle relaxation objectively and closed loop systems for muscle relaxant delivery have been used for some time. Perhaps because more simple administration schemes are also effective in providing muscle relaxation, these systems are rarely used.

Monitoring adequacy of anaesthesia

Monitoring the "depth" of anaesthesia is complex because anaesthesia itself is a complex process. Anaesthesia may be considered as a tetrad involving analgesia, hypnosis, suppression of autonomic responses, and muscle relaxation. While some of these aspects of anaesthesia can be readily monitored (e.g. HR, blood pressure, muscle relaxation), it is hypnosis or lack of awareness which is the most difficult to measure and also the most important to judge correctly. Movements by the patient, either gross and purposeful, small movements of the extremities or changes in respiratory rate or pattern are clear signals of inadequate anaesthesia. When muscle relaxant drugs are used, however, these signs are lost and there is a significant risk of the patient being aware during their operation but unable to communicate the fact. Although the neuromuscular blocking drugs do not abolish haemodynamic and other autonomic signs of light anaesthesia, these signs are non-specific and may be modified by fluid volume status and the use of other drugs, including anticholinergics, α and β receptor drugs, and opioid analgesics. Lack of intraoperative recall is currently the only definitive criterion of adequate anaesthesia. This is clearly a retrospective measure and is of no use during a procedure other than as an overall contribution to the "experience" of the anaesthetist. Furthermore, recall is subjective and there is evidence that patients may be aware intraoperatively but not recall this subsequently.

As long ago as 1937, Guedel described a variety of clinical signs reflecting the adequacy of ether anaesthesia. Although this was a substantial advance at the time, many of these signs are inappropriate for use with other anaesthetics and/or in the presence of muscle relaxants. The situation is further complicated by the use of various combinations of drugs to achieve the different components of the anaesthetic state, with consequently differing effects on various organ systems. Nevertheless, while the heart rate and blood pressure can be readily monitored and controlled with a variety of drugs and muscle relaxation tailored to individual needs (usually of the surgeon!), from the patient's point of view it is lack of awareness which constitutes "adequate" anaesthesia.

Awareness during anaesthesia

It is difficult to know how frequently awareness occurs in the clinical practice of anaesthesia, as many cases are not reported. In one published series where almost 63 000 patients were questioned after their anaesthetic, the incidence of awareness was approximately 12·4 per 10 000 anaesthetics.[10] In the past, many patients did not realise that awareness under anaesthesia was possible and attributed their experience to dreaming or imagination. As public "awareness" of this issue has increased, more cases have been reported[11] and these are more likely to result in legal action.

Between 1989 and 1990, awareness accounted for 12·2% of anaesthetic related legal claims sufficiently serious to require expert medical review.[11] Unfortunately, claims for awareness by National Health Service patients are now handled locally and national statistics are therefore not recorded. Statistics are available in the private health care sector, however, where claims for awareness currently comprise 15% of all anaesthetic related claims (excluding those for minor dental damage) (data from the Medical Defence Union).

Most cases of patient awareness occur when neuromuscular blocking drugs have been used. In the absence of these drugs, inadequate anaesthesia results in movements which are detected, allowing corrective action to be taken, before the patient becomes aware. Awareness is also associated with high dose opioid "anaesthesia" and is more common during emergency surgery, especially in haemodynamically unstable patients. In the past, it was common to use relatively "light" levels of anaesthesia during caesarean section in the mistaken belief that more profound anaesthesia would have adverse effects on the baby. As a result, awareness and recall were once quite common in this population. Better understanding of foetomaternal physiology has now reduced this problem with the realisation that inadequate anaesthesia causes stress in the mother which is transferred to her unborn child with harmful effects on both parties.

It is not possible to say whether or not awareness is more common with iv anaesthesia than with inhaled agents because neither the incidence of awareness nor the total number of iv and inhalational anaesthetics is known. One series reported five cases of awareness out of a total of 1727 total iv anaesthetics in which adequate patient followup was performed.[12] All these cases were due to a mixture of technical and human errors and all were considered avoidable. With the complex relationship between infusion rate over time and plasma anaesthetic concentration, as well as the inherent risks of infusion pump malfunction and misprogramming, extravasation of iv drug, and backflow of iv anaesthetic along a concurrently administered iv infusion line (fig 5.11), "Awareness under anaesthesia is a major threat with a total intravenous technique".[13] Some of these problems are preventable, however, with improved understanding of pharmacokinetic principles and more sophisticated infusion equipment.

Recall involves the patient being aware or conscious and remembering the event afterwards. It is also possible for a patient to be aware and obey commands during an operation, but subsequently to have no memory of this. This phenomenon has been studied by investigators using the isolated forearm technique (IFT). This involves the use of an arterial tourniquet to prevent muscle relaxants from reaching one of the patient's arms. If the patient is aware during anaesthesia, they can respond by moving the hand of the isolated arm. Using this technique, up to 40% of patients anaesthetised with N_2O moved their hand to command, although only

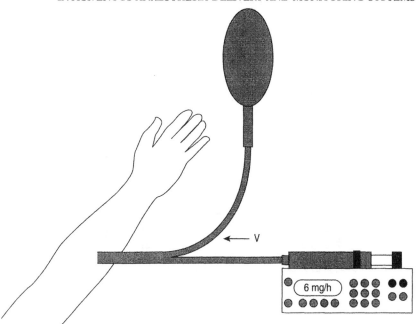

Fig 5.11 Diagram showing how an intravenous anaesthetic infused under high pressure may flow back up an attached infusion line, resulting in reduced drug delivery and the possibility of awareness. This backflow may be prevented by a non-return valve at point V or by administering fluids and intravenous drugs through separate intravenous cannulae

4–8% had subsequent recall.[14] Patients may also demonstrate learning or "implicit memory" under anaesthesia without demonstrating either awareness or recall. This may be demonstrated by patients "remembering" (when prompted) key words or aspects of a story conveyed to them during anaesthesia. There is some evidence that the use of positive, encouraging suggestions made during anaesthesia reduces postoperative analgesic requirements and may smooth and hasten recovery. It has also been suggested that memory of adverse comments or prognostic information may result in an unfavourable outcome such as psychosis or sleep disturbance. These findings are somewhat controversial and have not been consistently confirmed by other studies. It nevertheless seems prudent to prevent patients from "hearing" adverse comments during anaesthesia and it is not likely to do any harm to supply music or positive suggestions via headphones.

Measurements of anaesthetic adequacy

A variety of methods have been suggested for monitoring the adequacy of anaesthesia (table 5.3). Movement of the patient in response to surgery is

115

Table 5.3   Methods for assessing adequacy of anaesthesia

Method	Advantages	Disadvantages
Clinical signs		
Awareness	"Gold standard"	Retrospective
		May occur without recall
Purposeful movement	Reasonably reliable	Not totally reliable
	Usually obvious	Useless when muscle relaxants used
Respiratory rate and pattern	Reasonably reliable	Not totally reliable
		Useless when muscle relaxants used
Autonomic signs	Readily available	Very unreliable
(e.g. HR, BP, pupils, sweating)	Frequently used	Highly non-specific
EEG		
Raw signal	Relatively easy to monitor	Difficult to interpret
		Not independent of anaesthetic agent
Simple processed	Relatively easy to interpret	Need for special equipment
(e.g. CSA, SEF)		Not independent of anaesthetic agent
		Probably unreliable
Complex processed	Relatively easy to interpret	Need for special equipment
(e.g. BIS)	Promising; may be reliable	? independent of anaesthetic agent
		Needs further evaluation
Other techniques		
Facial muscles	Unaffected by muscle relaxants	Need for special equipment
	May be promising in the future	Needs further evaluation
Lower oesophageal contractility	None apparent	Need for special equipment
		Non-specific and unreliable
Evoked potentials	May be useful in the future	Need for special equipment
		Needs further evaluation

HR Heart rate; BP Blood pressure; CSA Compressed spectral array; SEF Spectral edge frequency; BIS Bispectral index a clear sign of inadequate anaesthesia. Movement (or lack of it) in response to a surgical incision is used as a measure of anaesthetic potency by determining the MAC of an anaesthetic vapour which prevents movement in response to this stimulus in 50% of subjects. Subsequently, a number of other MACs have been described. MAC-awake is the concentration which is required for loss of consciousness (lower than MAC), while MAC-BAR is the concentration needed to block haemodynamic responses to a painful stimulus and is the highest value of the three. Interestingly, prevention of movement by anaesthetics may be substantially mediated via the spinal cord. When the brain is perfused separately in experimental animals, a higher anaesthetic concentration is needed to prevent movement compared to perfusion of the body as a whole. This may explain the occasional reports of awareness when muscle relaxants were not used and patient movements were not observed.

In the absence of purposeful movement, it is common to use a variety of clinical signs to judge anaesthetic depth. These include cardiovascular parameters, respiratory rate and rhythm, muscle tone, ocular signs, lacrimation, and sweating (diaphoresis). Changes in heart rate and blood pressure are exceedingly non-specific and unreliable and may also vary with different anaesthetic agents. A variety of signs may be needed in order to increase the likelihood of detecting inadequate anaesthesia. For example, when systolic blood pressure, heart rate, movement, swallowing, coughing, grimacing, eye opening, lacrimation, flushing, and diaphoresis were monitored during alfentanil-N_2O anaesthesia, no single sign proved a consistent indicator of satisfactory anaesthesia.[15] Interpretation of haemodynamic signs is made more difficult by the differing ability of various anaesthetics and analgesics to produce tachycardia, bradycardia, and/or hypotension. Other clinical signs such as diaphoresis and lacrimation are also unreliable. Changes in these signs may not occur even in the presence of haemodynamic and motor responses, as well as in patients who subsequently report recall. Sweating is greatly affected by temperature changes, especially during cardiac surgery where active warming and cooling are both employed routinely. Similarly, eye signs are modified or lost after ocular operations or in the presence of opioids, atropine or other eye drops. For these reasons, attempts have been made to find a more specific and universally reliable indicator of anaesthetic depth.

Measurements from muscles not affected by neuromuscular blocking drugs have been evaluated. The facial muscles are relatively resistant to muscle relaxants, and voltages can be recorded from the frontalis, corrugator, zygomatic, and orbicularis oculi muscles using facial electromyography (FACE) and surface electrodes. It has been suggested that the pattern of muscle tension (e.g. grimace or smile) may be indicative of anaesthetic adequacy, although further evaluation is required. Lower oesophageal (esophageal) contractility (LEC) has also been evaluated as an

117

anaesthetic monitor.[16] Unfortunately, the pattern of LEC response appears to differ markedly from volatile to iv anaesthetics and is also influenced by anticholinergic drugs. Such fundamental problems mean that LEC is unlikely to become a clinically useful monitor of anaesthesia.

Many of the approaches to monitoring anaesthetic adequacy have involved some aspect of the EEG, either using raw signals or, more commonly, some processed form. The EEG is non-invasive and is a logical choice of anaesthetic monitor as the brain is clearly the primary site of action of general anaesthetics. The raw EEG is of limited use as it is a complex display of numerous signals which are difficult to interpret. In addition, different anaesthetics produce a variety of unique EEG patterns – not helpful in developing a universal monitor.

Processing the EEG begins with converting short sections of EEG signal (known as epochs) into digital form. The digitised EEG can then be mathematically transformed by a process known as Fourier analysis, which separates the complex signal of the EEG into a number of component sine waves, each of different amplitude but whose sum comprises the original EEG waveform.[17] The power spectrum can then be obtained from the relative amplitude of each frequency band (fig 5.12). The power spectrum of each processed EEG segment, or epoch, can be displayed graphically. More information can be given if a number of consecutive epochs are displayed closely above each other, producing a compressed spectral array (CSA), which produces a characteristic "hill and valley" pattern (fig 5.12). The "hills" of the CSA represent those frequencies of the EEG where the greatest amplitude (or power) is located. An alternative form of presentation is to calculate the frequency below which 95% of the total power is present, which is known as the spectral edge frequency (SEF).[18] The greatest advantage of the SEF is that it is a single number, which has long been thought to correlate with adequate anaesthesia. Many conflicting studies have been performed, however, suggesting that SEF does or does not correlate well with haemodynamic responses or purposeful movement.

Conventional EEG power analysis does not retain information on the phase relationship between the different components of the EEG. Bispectral analysis (BIS) is another method of EEG analysis which allows relationships between the phases of different frequencies to be examined[19] and may better represent the information contained within the original EEG (fig 5.13). BIS has been shown to predict movement in response to skin incision during isoflurane/oxygen anaesthesia,[19] as well as with propofol/alfentanil and isoflurane/alfentanil.[20] BIS does not appear to be independent of anaesthetic technique, however, with different responses being obtained depending on whether hypnotics or analgesics are used as the primary anaesthetic agent.[20] This may prove to be a potential problem with BIS monitoring or may simply reflect the fact that hypnotics and analgesics have different clinical effects. While movement represents a

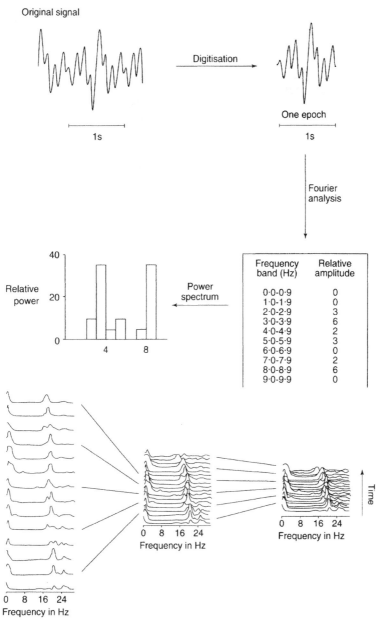

Fig 5.12 Diagram showing EEG power spectrum analysis. The original signal (top left) is digitised into a one second section (epoch), which then undergoes Fourier analysis to derive the amplitude of each frequency band from which the power is then plotted as a histogram. Subsequently, consecutive epochs of analysis are plotted above each other and stacked closer and closer together to form the characteristic "hill and valley" pattern. Reproduced with permission[17]

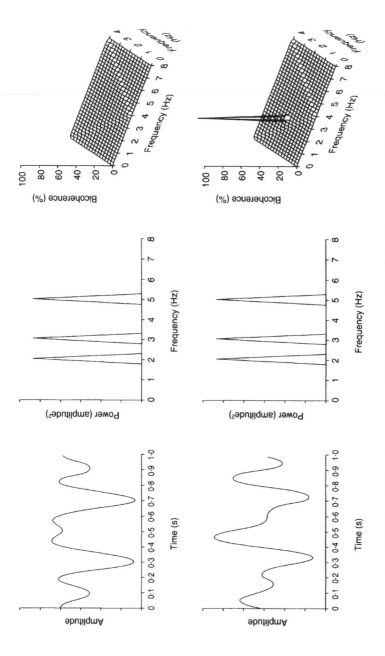

Fig 5.13 Comparison of EEG analysis using power analysis and bispectral analysis. The upper panel shows a simple EEG comprising three sine waves of 2 Hz, 3 Hz, and 5 Hz with no phase relationship and the resulting power spectrum and bispectrum. The lower panel shows another EEG where the 2 Hz and 3 Hz waves produce a harmonic at 5 Hz. Although this EEG looks different, it has an identical power spectrum to the first, but the bispectrum clearly shows the interaction of the 2 Hz and 3 Hz components. Reproduced with permission[19]

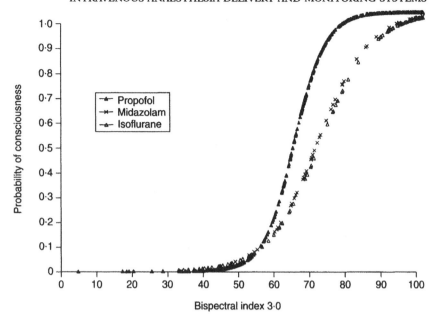

Fig 5.14 Relationship between bispectral index and probability of a positive response to verbal command in volunteers receiving a range of concentrations of propofol, midazolam or isoflurane. Note that the bispectral index corresponding to a 50% probability of a response to propofol (approximately 62) is lower than that for isoflurane and midazolam (approximately 70). Reproduced with permission[21]

response to a noxious stimulus, it may reflect a different aspect of brain function to awareness under anaesthesia. Attempts have therefore been made to correlate BIS with sedation, especially at that level of sedation at which subjects move from consciousness to unconsciousness. At present, BIS has been shown to correlate remarkably well with responsiveness to verbal command during sedation in volunteers with a range of sedative agents,[21] although again, the values recorded varied somewhat between different sedative agents (fig 5.14).

An alternative to using passive EEG data is the acquisition of evoked responses. As the auditory system appears to be the least susceptible to the effects of general anaesthesia, most efforts have concentrated on the auditory evoked response. A simple auditory stimulus (e.g. a "click") is applied and the EEG is recorded immediately afterwards from a variety of anatomical areas. A variety of responses are recognised, including the brainstem response, which is the first to occur, followed by the middle latency response originating within the thalamus and auditory cortex and finally the late cortical response from the frontal cortex (fig 5.15). Most anaesthetic and analgesic drugs have little effect on the brainstem response, whereas the mid latency response shows a dose related effect with a variety

121

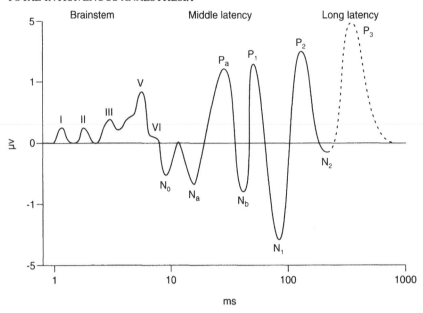

Fig 5.15 The auditory evoked response resulting from a sound stimulus. The initial waves (I to VI) originate in the brainstem, the middle latency waves originate in the thalamus and auditory cortex while the long latency waves originate in other cortical areas. Reproduced with permission[23]

of anaesthetics (fig 5.16). The pattern of mid latency responses appears similar with different anaesthetics. Interestingly, these changes are not observed with high dose fentanyl, consistent with the high incidence of awareness associated with this technique. Auditory evoked potentials may be a useful tool for assessing anaesthetic adequacy in the future.

Controlling the stress response

Surgery produces a complex "stress" response, manifested by a number of endocrine, haemodynamic, metabolic, and inflammatory changes. Initially, catecholamine release increases gluconeogenesis, mobilises fat and protein, and causes sodium and water retention. This is followed by the release of steroid and peptide hormones, producing a sustained catabolic reaction with baseline metabolic conditions not being restored for several days or weeks. This stress response may increase the incidence of perioperative cardiovascular, pulmonary, and gastrointestinal morbidity and even mortality. While several studies have investigated the ability of inhalational, intravenous or regional anaesthetics to modify this stress reaction, few have examined clinical outcome following such interventions. It is currently believed that modifying the stress response will reduce

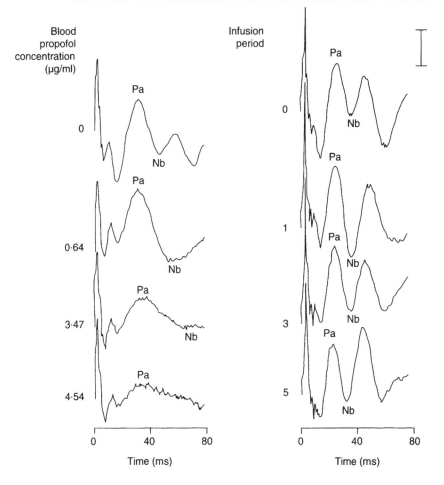

Fig 5.16 Brainstem and early cortical evoked responses to increasing doses of propofol (left panel) or saline (right panel). Note no significant change in the brainstem response, but decreasing amplitude and increasing latency in the early cortical response (Pa and Nb waves) following increasing propofol concentration. In contrast, saline has no effect on any of the responses. Reproduced with permission[24]

morbidity and mortality associated with anaesthesia and surgery, although there are very few data to support this contention.

The effect of anaesthesia on the stress response

Although deeper levels of the volatile anaesthetics can reduce levels of stress hormones compared to relatively "light" anaesthesia, inhaled anaesthetics do not appear to completely block the stress response. The effects of the intravenous hypnotics appear to vary from one agent to

123

another. For example, the barbiturates have only limited metabolic and endocrine effects, with some reduction in hyperglycaemia but little effect on the adrenocortical response.

Etomidate can inhibit the adrenocortical response to surgery, but has no effect on the catecholamine response. The effect of etomidate on the adrenocortical response is due to inhibition of an enzyme (11β hydroxylase) required for cortisol synthesis, rather than any antinociceptive effect. Furthermore, this inhibition of cortisol synthesis by etomidate is believed to be associated with increased (rather than decreased) mortality, at least when used for sedation in the ICU (see chapter 3).

Compared to thiopentone, propofol appears to produce a greater reduction in ACTH and cortisol secretion. In addition, propofol appears to be equally or more effective in controlling acute haemodynamic and hormonal responses compared to opioid analgesics.[22]

Midazolam and other benzodiazepines reduce the adrenal response to surgery by decreasing ACTH secretion, as well as by the production of several cytokines which have been implicated in the stress response.

Despite the profound analgesia provided by ketamine, its use is associated with hypertension and significant increases in ACTH, cortisol, and prolactin. These effects of ketamine are due to direct sympathetic stimulation, inhibition of reuptake of catecholamines, and modification of the pituitary–adrenal axis, resulting in the release of ACTH and aldosterone. Concomitant administration of midazolam may prevent the rise in catecholamine levels, but had less effect on the other stress hormones. The use of other hypnotic agents (e.g. propofol) with ketamine may have a more beneficial effect on the stress response. The effect of both R(−) and S(+) ketamine on stress hormone levels does not appear to differ from that of the racemic mixture.

The opioid analgesics are the drugs most commonly used to attenuate the stress response. At high doses (e.g. fentanyl 50–100 µg/kg), there is a substantial reduction in the release of a variety of stress hormones, including adrenaline, noradrenaline, dopamine, cortisol, growth hormone, aldosterone, endorphins, and vasopressin. Lower doses of opioids also appear able to reduce the surgical stress response, especially when administered with other anaesthetic agents. Indeed, the use of lower opioid doses appears just as effective at suppressing hormone release, but with a lower incidence of adverse effects such as prolonged ventilatory depression and muscle rigidity. When a balanced (opioid and hypnotic) technique is used, however, no difference has been shown between increasing the opioid dose and administering additional hypnotic in terms of their ability to effectively treat a hypertensive response.[22]

How do the opioids reduce the stress response? In part, they reduce nociceptive stimulation of higher centres by modifying ascending and descending pain pathways and, perhaps, also by a peripheral analgesic effect. In addition, the opioids have effects on a variety of neurohormonal systems, probably by interaction with natural endorphins. The stress response can also be reduced by other drugs which modify nociceptive input, such as the α_2 agonists (see chapter 3). For example, perioperative therapy with clonidine has been shown to significantly reduce circulating catecholamines during cardiac and major vascular surgery. Although the NSAIDs are effective analgesics and also have antipyretic properties (increased temperature appears to increase hypothalamo-pituitary-adreno-cortical activity), their perioperative use does not appear to significantly modify the stress response.

Summary

Although iv anaesthetics can be administered using minimal equipment, more controllable and reliable anaesthesia results from the use of infusions. Fixed rate infusions, incorporating a small number of predetermined steps, can achieve relatively constant plasma levels of drug without sophisticated technology. In contrast, variable rate infusions allow the level of anaesthesia to be adjusted in relation to the individual levels of stimulus and response. TCI may allow these two approaches to be combined by delivering a stable plasma concentration which can then be adjusted up or down to another stable concentration depending upon the clinical response. At present, the ability of TCI systems to maintain a stable concentration in a wide range of patients is in some doubt. This may improve with further refinement of the pharmacokinetic models for a greater range of patient groups and a larger selection of drugs. In the meantime, the further evaluation of these systems to determine whether they improve our ability to deliver anaesthesia compared to alternative means is a clear priority. Drug delivery, either by manual, semiautomatic or even fully automatic means, will no doubt improve if a reliable and universally acceptable monitor of the anaesthetic state can be developed.

Unfortunately, despite a variety of interesting developments in interpretation of the EEG, there is as yet no simple, non-invasive, reliable, and easy to use "depth of anaesthesia" monitor which will provide real time predictive information with a wide variety of anaesthetic drugs and techniques. At present, the anaesthetist has to rely on experience in judging the efficacy of anaesthesia, aided by an assessment of a variety of clinical responses in relation to differing stimuli. Information from the processed EEG can now be added to this array of information, but is not yet a substitute for these valuable clinical skills.

The alterations in haemodynamic parameters which we commonly observe as part of our routine patient monitoring are only one manifestation of the stress response which invariably accompanies surgery. It is clear that a variety of iv hypnotic, analgesic, and adjunctive drugs (e.g.

125

barbiturates, etomidate, propofol, benzodiazepines, opioids, and α_2 agonists) can modify the stress response to surgical stimuli. Few, if any, drugs or techniques currently in use can totally prevent this response, however, and there is little clear evidence that any one drug (or drug type) is significantly more effective than another. Indeed, there is no evidence to prove that modifying the stress response has any beneficial effect on clinical outcome or that there is any difference between a balanced or total intravenous anaesthetic technique with respect to patient outcome after surgery. This aspect will be discussed further in the next chapter.

1 White PF. Clinical uses of intravenous anesthetic and analgesic infusions. *Anesth Analg* 1989;68:161–71.
2 Roberts FL, Dixon J, Lewis GTR, Tackley RM, Prys-Roberts C. Induction and maintenance of propofol anaesthesia. A manual infusion scheme. *Anaesthesia* 1988;43(Supplement):14–17.
3 Tackley RM, Lewis GT, Prys Roberts C, *et al.* Computer controlled infusion of propofol. *Br J Anaesth* 1989;62:46–53.
4 Chaudhri S, White M, Kenny GN. Induction of anaesthesia with propofol using a target-controlled infusion system. *Anaesthesia* 1992;47:551–3.
5 Coetzee JF, Glen JB, Wium CA, Boshoff L. Pharmacokinetic model selection for target controlled infusions of propofol. Assessment of three parameter sets. *Anesthesiology* 1995;82:1328–45.
6 Shafer SL. Advances in propofol pharmacokinetics and pharmacodynamics. *J Clin Anesth* 1993;5(supplement 1):14S–21S.
7 Doyle E, McFadzean W, Morton NS. I.V. anaesthesia with propofol using a target-controlled infusion system: comparison with inhalation anaesthesia for general surgical procedures in children. *Br J Anaesth* 1993;70:542–5.
8 Davidson JA, McLeod AD, Howie JC, White M, Kenny GN. Effective concentration 50 for propofol with and without 67% nitrous oxide. *Acta Anaesthesiol Scand* 1993;37:458–64.
9 Irwin MG, Thompson N, Kenny GNC. Patient-maintained propofol sedation. Assessment of a target-controlled infusion system. *Anaesthesia* 1997;52:525–30.
10 Cohen MM, Duncan PG, Pope WDB, Wolkenstein C. A survey of 112,000 anaesthetics at one teaching hospital (1975–83). *Can Anaesth Soc J* 1986;33:22–31.
11 Aitkenhead AR. Risk management in anaesthesia. *J Med Defence Union* 1991;4:86–90.
12 Sandin R, Nordström O. Awareness during total i.v. anaesthesia. *Br J Anaesth* 1993;71:782–7.
13 Mallon JS, Edelist G. Total intravenous anesthesia (editorial). *Can J Anaesth* 1990;37:279–81.
14 Russell IF. Balanced anesthesia: does it anesthetize? *Anesth Analg* 1985;64:941–2.
15 Ausems ME, Hug CC Jr, Stanski DR, Burm AGL. Plasma concentrations of alfentanil required to supplement nitrous oxide anesthesia for general surgery. *Anesthesiology* 1986;65:362–73.
16 Watcha MF, White PF. Failure of lower esophageal contractility to predict patient movement in children anesthetized with halothane and nitrous oxide. *Anesthesiology* 1989;71:664–8.
17 Levy WJ, Shapiro HM, Maruchak G, Meathe E. Automated EEG processing for intraoperative monitoring: a comparison of techniques. *Anesthesiology* 1980;53:223–36.
18 Rampil IJ, Holzer JA, Quest DO, Rosenbaum SH, Correll JW. Prognostic value of computerized EEG analysis during carotid endarterectomy. *Anesth Analg* 1983;62:186–92.
19 Sebel PS, Bowles SM, Saini V, Chamoun N. EEG bispectrum predicts movement during thiopental/isoflurane anesthesia. *J Clin Monit* 1995;11:83–91.
20 Vernon JM, Lang E, Sebel PS, Manberg P. Prediction of movement using bispectral electroencephalographic analysis during propofol/alfentanil or isoflurane/alfentanil anes-

thesia. *Anesth Analg* 1995;**80**:780–5.

21 Glass PSA, Bloom M, Kearse L, *et al.* Bispectral analysis measures sedation and memory effects of propofol, midazolam, isoflurane, and alfentanil in healthy volunteers. *Anesthesiology* 1997;**86**:836–47.

22 Monk TG, Ding Y, White PF. Total intravenous anesthesia: effects of opioid versus hypnotic supplementation on autonomic responses and recovery. *Anesth Analg* 1992;**75**:798–804.

23 Ghoneim MM, Block RI. Learning and consciousness during general anaesthesia. *Anesthesiology* 1992;**76**:279–305.

24 Thornton C, Konieczko KM, Knight AB, *et al.* Effect of propofol on the auditory evoked response and oesophageal contractility. *Br J Anaesth* 1989;**63**:411–7.

6: Advantages and disadvantages of intravenous anaesthesia

Introduction

Although intravenous anaesthesia is increasing in popularity, the technique is still used infrequently for routine anaesthetic maintenance. In contrast, iv anaesthesia is almost universally used in some special areas of practice, such as cardiac anaesthesia. This has occurred because a clear advantage for iv anaesthetics over inhaled agents is seen to exist in this specific situation. Any technique will inevitably be associated with its own advantages and disadvantages. Inhaled anaesthesia has the advantage of familiarity, so if it is to be displaced by alternative techniques, there must be some benefit to outweigh the inconvenience of a change in practice.

This chapter will review the relative advantages and disadvantages of iv anaesthetic techniques, in relation to both other iv techniques and inhaled anaesthesia. Consideration will be given to the organ toxicity of the different drugs and to the impact of various anaesthetic techniques on a range of postoperative patient outcomes.

Because iv anaesthetic drugs are more specific than their inhaled counterparts, it is usually necessary to administer a combination of drugs and so interactions are almost inevitable. The mechanisms of a variety of interactions will be examined, as will a number of commonly encountered and clinically important interactions. Consideration will be given to how drug interactions may have both advantageous and disadvantageous effects.

Organ and tissue toxicity

Direct toxicity resulting from anaesthesia is uncommon with any of the anaesthetics (iv and inhaled) currently in use. Nevertheless, the volatile agents are associated with a few uncommon forms of toxicity which can be avoided by the use of iv anaesthetics.

Malignant hyperpyrexia

Malignant hyperpyrexia (MH) occurs in individuals with a genetically determined abnormality of the sarcolemma or sarcoplasmic reticulum. Manifestation of the disease requires a susceptible individual and a trigger agent. MH is characterised by hypermetabolism, increased oxygen consumption, increased carbon dioxide production causing respiratory acidosis, muscle contractures, and a rapid increase in temperature. If untreated, the condition is usually fatal, but recognition of the early signs (with removal of trigger agents) and treatment with dantrolene will usually terminate an attack. Overall, the incidence of MH ranges from 1 in 6000 to 1 in 200 000. All the volatile anaesthetics can trigger MH, whereas most of the iv hypnotics and the opioids appear safe and can be used in MH susceptible individuals. The non-depolarising relaxant suxamethonium is also a potent trigger, however, although the non-depolarising relaxants are not.

"Halothane hepatitis"

Fulminant, massive hepatic necrosis occasionally occurs following halothane exposure. Between 1978 and 1985, 84 reports of serious hepatotoxicity were received by the Committee on Safety of Medicines. In patients where a clear history of halothane exposure was available, mortality was close to 40% and appeared to increase if patients had multiple previous exposures to halothane. It is now known that halothane undergoes extensive ($>20\%$) metabolism to trifluroacetic acid (TFA). TFA can subsequently react with hepatic proteins to produce a new complex, to which certain individuals mount an immune response. Subsequent exposure to halothane or another anaesthetic producing similar protein conjugates can trigger immune mediated hepatic necrosis. Although halothane undergoes a greater degree of metabolism than other volatile anaesthetics, isoflurane and desflurane can also produce small quantities of TFA, while enflurane produces an intermediary which can also react with liver proteins to produce immunologically identical complexes (fig 6.1). The likelihood of hepatic injury is related to the degree to which the anaesthetics are metabolised (enflurane $\approx 2\%$, isoflurane $\approx 0\cdot2\%$, and desflurane $\approx 0\cdot02\%$). It is unlikely that the newer volatile anaesthetics undergo sufficient metabolism to initiate antibody production, although they may trigger hepatitis in a previously sensitised individual and there are case reports of hepatic necrosis following enflurane, isoflurane, and desflurane. Although iv anaesthetics are extensively metabolised, none of the breakdown products produce crossreacting protein conjugates (or other known immunogenic complexes) and therefore do not produce hepatitis. Sevoflurane also avoids this risk as it has a very different structure from the other halogenated ethers (fig 6.1) and does not form hepatic protein conjugates, despite a moderate degree of metabolism ($\approx 7\%$).

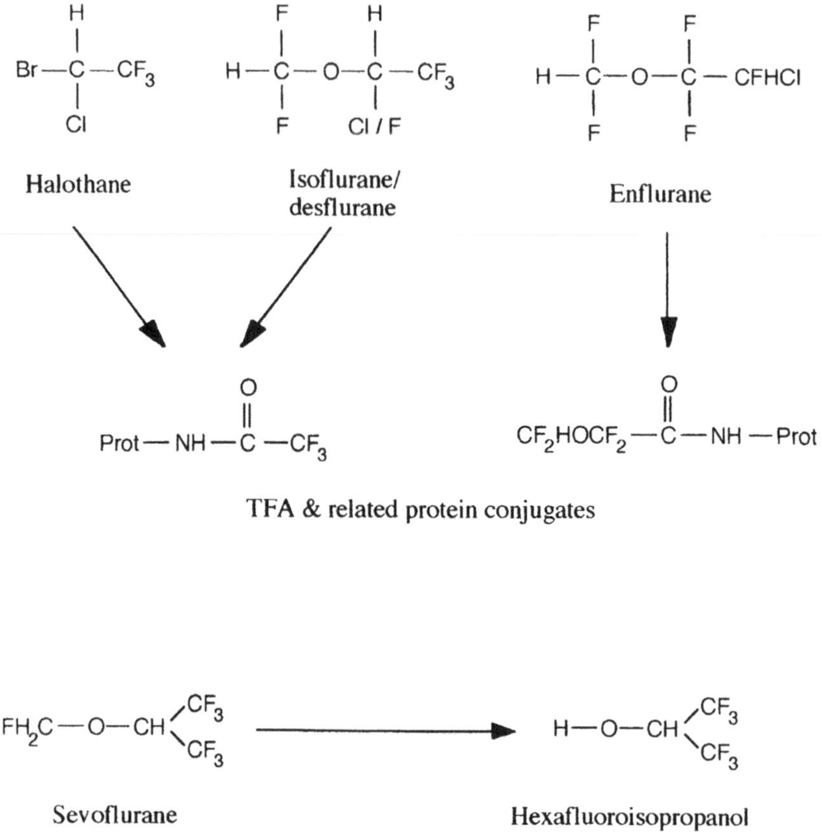

Fig 6.1 Metabolic pathways of halothane, isoflurane, and desflurane to trifluro-acetic acid (TFA) protein conjugates, enflurane to related protein conjugates and sevoflurane to hexafluoroisopropanol

Fluoride toxicity

Metabolism of the inhalational anaesthetic methoxyflurane produced significant amounts of inorganic fluoride ions which often produced renal damage, especially high output renal failure. The likelihood of renal damage was initially thought to increase if plasma fluoride levels exceeded 50 μmol/l, although this is now known to be too simplistic a relationship. Methoxyflurane is no longer available, although two of the current inhaled anaesthetics, enflurane and sevoflurane, also produce fluoride. Enflurane yields less fluoride than either methoxyflurane and sevoflurane, yet it can produce detectable (but subclinical) impairment of renal function with prolonged use. Enflurane is probably best avoided for prolonged cases or in the presence of preexisting renal failure. Sevoflurane produces more fluoride

130

than enflurane, yet has not been shown to cause renal impairment, even in patients with poor renal function.[1] This is probably because it is defluorinated mainly in the liver rather than the kidney and also because it is rapidly eliminated. Nevertheless, our total experience with sevoflurane is less than that with enflurane. None of the iv anaesthetics or analgesics produce inorganic fluoride following their metabolism.

Soda lime breakdown products

As the cost of inhaled anaesthesia is primarily flow dependent, there are considerable advantages to the use of low fresh gas flows. A variety of inhaled anaesthetics can interact with soda lime (and other CO_2 absorbants) to produce potential toxins. If soda lime is allowed to completely dry out (by flushing with oxygen for several hours), carbon monoxide may be produced by breakdown of enflurane, isoflurane, and desflurane (but not halothane or sevoflurane). Levels of several thousand parts per million (ppm) can be produced from completely dry soda lime. Such complete dryness of soda lime should not be achieved during normal use, however, and there are currently no reports of patient injury from this cause.

Halothane is significantly degraded by soda lime. One of the breakdown products, 2-bromo-2-chloro-1,1-difluoroethylene (BCDFE), is toxic in mice at levels of about 250 ppm. The toxicity of BCDFE in humans is not known, but levels achieved clinically are only about 5 ppm, 50 times less than those toxic to animals. Sevoflurane is also degraded by soda lime, producing an olefin known as compound A. Compound A is lethal to rats at levels of about 1000 ppm. Again, levels produced clinically are substantially below this (20–30 ppm), although there is concern that renal damage may occur in rats at levels above 50 ppm. While this is close to clinically relevant concentrations, renal damage has not been detected in humans to date.[1]

Intravenous anaesthetics do not come into contact with soda lime and so cannot undergo degradation. Furthermore, when anaesthesia is maintained using iv drugs, there is little advantage to using very low fresh gas flows. The modest heat and moisture conservation can be achieved in other ways, while the cost of volatile anaesthetics and atmospheric pollution are no longer issues. Soda lime can therefore be easily avoided during iv anaesthesia.

Other toxicity

Toxicity associated with iv anaesthetics is rare. Certain forms of porphyria may be exacerbated by a wide range of drugs. Barbiturates, benzodiazepines, and steroid anaesthetics are all contraindicated. Several iv anaesthetics (e.g. propofol, etomidate, ketamine) are safe, however, as are most of the inhaled anaesthetics. Hepatic and renal toxicity may also relate to blood flow to these organs. Under normal circumstances, most iv anaesthetics cause moderate reductions in blood flow, although they may have greater effects in disease states and during hypovolaemia. In practice, large scale retrospective surveys have failed to demonstrate any significant differences in overall toxicity and organ damage between inhaled and iv anaesthetics.

Drug interactions

As has already been stated (chapter 2), anaesthesia consists of a tetrad of hypnosis, analgesia, autonomic suppression, and muscle relaxation. Compared to volatile anaesthetics, the intravenous agents are generally more specific for each of these activities. Providing a complete, or balanced, anaesthetic necessarily involves the administration of two or more drugs in combination to provide these various components and the possibility of drug interaction therefore exists. Whereas the interaction between two volatile agents is approximately additive (i.e. 60% of the MAC of one agent combined with 40% of the MAC of another agent will produce the same effect as one MAC of either agent alone), the interaction between intravenous drugs (or between inhalational and intravenous anaesthetics) results in complex drug interactions which are not easily predicted. This is because the intravenous hypnotics, analgesics, anxiolytics, and sympatholytics all have different receptors and mechanisms of action within the CNS. Interactions may take three forms. The effects of the drugs may simply be additive, as is generally the case with volatile anaesthetics. Synergy is said to occur when the effect of the drug combination is greater than that achieved by the sum of the two components given alone. Antagonism is observed when the effect of the combination is less than the sum of the components. Interactions may be beneficial if they increase desirable effects (or reduce adverse events) and detrimental if the converse situation occurs.

Mechanisms of interaction

Interactions between drugs may occur for a variety of reasons.

1. *Physicochemical*: the two drugs are incompatible when mixed together, for example, because of pH differences. This may prevent the administration of drug mixtures from the same syringe, but rarely causes a problem when drugs are sequentially administered into an intravenous cannula. Flushing the line or administration into a fast running infusion further reduces problems.

2. *Pharmacokinetic*: one drug alters the distribution or metabolism of another drug or modifies protein binding, thereby altering the plasma concentration of active unbound drug. For example, a reduction in cardiac output caused by one drug may reduce redistribution of a second drug, thereby increasing its plasma concentration.

3. *Pharmacodynamic*: may result from alteration of the receptor sensitivity of one drug by another or by the production of complementary (or antagonistic) effects at different receptor sites or by different mechanisms.

Assessment of drug interactions

The effect of combining two agents is measured by preparing dose–response curves for each individual agent and then comparing combinations using isobolographic analysis.[2] An isobole diagram plots the ED_{50} for each drug alone on the x and y axes, respectively (fig 6.2). These are then connected by a straight line which indicates those combinations of the two drugs which would have the same effect if the interaction between them were simply additive. If the actual point representing the combination

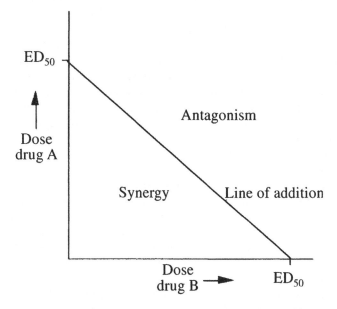

Fig 6.2 Simple isobologram. The ED_{50}s of drugs A and B are plotted and joined by a straight line. The doses of drugs A and B which, in combination, represent the ED_{50} are also plotted. If this point falls above (or to the right of) the line, the drug combination is antagonistic, if the point is below (or to the left of) the line, the combination is synergistic and if the point falls on the line, the effect of the combination is purely additive

resulting in ED_{50} falls below or to the left of this line, synergism is inferred, whereas a point above or to the right indicates antagonism.

Clinically important interactions

Midazolam interacts synergistically with the barbiturates, propofol, and the opioids. These interactions are all bidirectional, in that small doses of midazolam potentiate hypnotic and opioid effects and small doses of hypnotics or opioids also potentiate the benzodiazepine effects of midazolam. Both propofol and the barbiturates modify the binding of benzodiazepines to their receptor. These interactions are extremely powerful. For example, one tenth the ED_{50} dose of midazolam (0.02 mg/kg) can virtually halve the ED_{90} dose of thiopentone or propofol and can reduce the ED_{50} of alfentanil by almost 80%. One major advantage of these interactions is that total drug doses are substantially decreased, which can reduce costs. Furthermore, the degree of interpatient variability in anaesthetic induction dose is apparently reduced, making the induction requirements more predictable, reducing drug wastage, and further reducing costs.

These synergistic interactions may also have adverse effects. For example, there is a synergistic increase in ventilatory depression when combinations of opioids and midazolam are used. A dose of fentanyl insufficient to cause apnoea but which produced haemoglobin oxygen desaturation ($\leqslant 90\%$) in 50% of volunteers resulted in apnoea (no respiratory effort for $\geqslant 15$ s) in 50% of subjects and desaturation in 95% when administered along with a dose of midazolam which produced no measurable respiratory effects when given alone (fig 6.3). Such interactions have been responsible for fatalities when opioid-benzodiazepine combinations are used for sedation (e.g. for endoscopy). Similarly, the combination of benzodiazepines and opiates results in more profound hypotension compared to the use of either drug alone.

A number of other important drug interactions are simply additive. This is the case when combining volatile anaesthetics or using these drugs with N_2O. Intravenous examples include the interaction of ketamine with thiopentone, propofol or midazolam and the interaction of propofol with opioid analgesics. Multiple drug interactions are also possible. For example, midazolam, opioids, and barbiturates all interact synergistically to reduce induction doses. Similarly, there is a synergistic interaction between opioids and benzodiazepines combined with an additive effect of propofol when these three types of drug are used together. In addition to a considerable reduction in induction doses, this combination can result in an accelerated onset of action compared to the use of an individual drug, improved haemodynamic stability (even with early tracheal intubation) and improved control of intraocular and intracranial pressure. A ceiling effect may also be observed. For example, small doses of opioid analgesics reduce the propofol induction requirements, although there is no significant additional effect above a plasma concentration of approximately 3–4 ng/ml for fentanyl or 100–150 ng/ml for alfentanil. Use of a low opioid dose will therefore achieve the optimal reduction in propofol dose while minimising side effects.

Outcome studies

Outcome after general anaesthesia may mean many things. Clearly, survival is a major, fundamentally important endpoint. In the early days of iv anaesthesia (e.g. the casualties at Pearl Harbor), use of inappropriately high doses in inadequately resuscitated patients produced a high mortality which was incorrectly attributed to the drug and technique.[4] Later, when iv anaesthesia was "reinvented" in the form of neurolept anaesthesia, it was associated with substantially lower mortality compared to alternative,

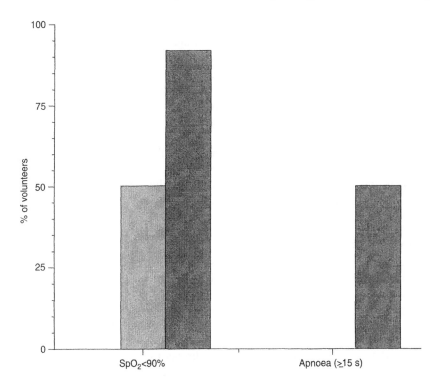

Fig 6.3   Percentage of volunteers experiencing haemoglobin oxygen desaturation (≤ 90%) or apnoea (no respiratory efforts for ≥ 15 s) after midazolam 50 μg/kg (open bars), fentanyl 2 μg/kg (lighter shade bars) or both drugs in combination (darker shade bars). Data from[3] with permission

135

concurrently available techniques. Since these early days, the overall mortality from anaesthesia has been reduced substantially from 1 in 1000 in 1944 to 1 in 250 000 by 1986.[5] All our modern anaesthetic techniques appear very safe and it is virtually impossible to distinguish small differences in mortality with one technique compared to another against such a background of apparent safety.

Similarly, it is difficult to evaluate any long term effects of anaesthesia on either the final response to surgical intervention or overall subsequent wellbeing of the recipient. With prolonged follow up, multiple other factors play a part in overall outcome and it would be virtually impossible to study sufficient numbers of patients in a rigidly controlled investigation designed to eliminate most other confounding variables. There is currently no evidence to suggest that iv anaesthesia results in any improved long term outcome compared to volatile based techniques, although there is a similar lack of evidence indicating a less favourable outcome.

Other measures of outcome are important too. In the short term, patients may appreciate a rapid and clearheaded recovery from anaesthesia. Day case patients may prefer an earlier return to their families. These are certainly major goals of day surgery, although there is little evidence to indicate what patients actually do want, as opposed to what their anaesthetists feel is good for them. Patients are certainly concerned about pain, as well as about adverse effects, especially PONV. A final measure of outcome is the total cost to society. Society wants cost effective health care, that is, it wants either improved health care for the same cost or to maintain healthcare standards at reduced costs.

Cost effective analysis must take into account all direct costs of drugs and techniques, but must also include indirect costs from recovery room and inpatient stay, as well as costs resulting from the need to treat adverse reactions. Finally, the overall cost to society from time away from work or disability must also be included.

Recovery after anaesthesia

One of the easiest outcomes to assess is emergence or early awakening after anaesthesia. It is implied (although by no means proven) that more rapid emergence will be associated with earlier return of protective reflexes and therefore greater safety. With the availability of skilled recovery staff and the continued use of airway support (via endotracheal tube [ETT] or laryngeal mask airway [LMA]), however, this may not be true. It is also suggested that more rapid awakening facilitates more efficient use of the operating room. Again, this may not be the case if care of the recovering patient is devolved to recovery room staff. Faster recovery may decrease costs if it reduces the time spent in the recovery room or if it permits earlier discharge of day case patients. Even those savings are heavily dependent upon how recovery room time is calculated and charged. Ultimately, financial benefits may only result from major changes in staffing policies. In practice, when a variety of anaesthetic techniques are compared for their effect on recovery, the differences are not that marked.

Early investigations, comparing propofol TIVA with "traditional" techniques comprising induction with thiopentone and maintenance with a volatile anaesthetic, have consistently demonstrated faster awakening and frequently also shown earlier discharge with propofol (table 6.1). When anaesthesia is induced with propofol and maintained with either propofol or a volatile anaesthetic, as is now common in day case practice, these differences are much less apparent (table 6.2). Indeed, the availability of the less soluble anaesthetic vapours, sevoflurane and desflurane, has tended to result in improved recovery compared to propofol TIVA, especially when the inhaled agents are also used for induction of anaesthesia.[6,7] Differences between anaesthetics become less apparent with increasing time. It is not surprising, therefore, that few studies have demonstrated differences in late recovery events (e.g. return to work after surgery). Following breast biopsy, women receiving a propofol anaesthetic were discharged earlier and returned to work half a day earlier (1.5 ± 0.1 versus 2.0 ± 0.1 days) compared to a group receiving a thiopentone-isoflurane anaesthetic.[8] In contrast, when anaesthesia was induced with propofol, no differences in a variety of performance tests could be demonstrated four hours after oral surgery between patients receiving propofol or enflurane for maintenance of anaesthesia.[9]

Hospital discharge times were also similar following major abdominal surgery with propofol-fentanyl compared to a group receiving isoflurane-fentanyl, although recovery of subjective control and social orientation were improved seven days after surgery in the TIVA group.[10] One area where TIVA (at least with propofol) appears to have an undisputed advantage is in the reduction of postoperative nausea and vomiting (PONV). Many factors influence the incidence of PONV aside from the anaesthetic technique, including unavoidable factors such as gender, previous history, and type of surgical operation. Nevertheless, propofol is consistently associated with a reduced incidence of PONV compared to alternative anaesthetics. This effect is noticeable after even an induction dose, but is most marked when propofol is used for maintenance of anaesthesia. For example, following maintenance of anaesthesia with isoflurane, the incidence of nausea (requiring treatment) was 44%, compared to 19% in a comparable group receiving a propofol infusion.[11] The incidence of PONV following sevoflurane may be more comparable to that observed with propofol, however.[6]

Following major abdominal surgery, propofol was associated with faster awakening and less PONV in the first two postoperative hours compared to the use of isoflurane for anaesthetic maintenance.[12] These apparent advantages in the early postoperative period were not reflected in a reduced

Table 6.1 Comparison of propofol for induction and maintenance of outpatient anaesthesia with "conventional" intravenous-inhalation techniques

Reference	Propofol administration[+]	Comparative group		Principal findings[*]
		Induction	Maintenance	
Ding et al., 1993	VRI	Thiopentone	Enflurane	Faster emergence; later recovery equal
Millar & Jewkes, 1988	IB	Thiopentone	Enflurane	Faster emergence and discharge
Price et al., 1988	VRI	Thiopentone	Enflurane	Faster recovery at 15–30 min
Puttick & Rosen, 1988	IB	Thiopentone	Halothane	Faster emergence and discharge
Sear et al., 1988	VRI	Thiopentone	Halothane	Faster emergence
Doze et al., 1988	VRI	Thiopentone	Isoflurane	Faster emergence and ambulation
Gold et al., 1989	FRI	Thiopentone	Isoflurane	Earlier discharge from recovery room
Korttila et al., 1990	FRI	Thiopentone	Isoflurane	Faster emergence and discharge
Lim & Low, 1992	FRI	Thiopentone	Isoflurane	Faster emergence and ambulation
Marais et al., 1989	Not reported	Thiopentone	Isoflurane	Faster emergence and discharge
Sung et al., 1991	VRI	Thiopentone	Isoflurane	Faster recovery and discharge

[+] VRI Variable rate infusion; FRI Fixed rate infusion; IB Intermittent bolus doses
[*] Findings are expressed with respect to the propofol group
Modified with permission from [14]

Table 6.2 Comparison of propofol for induction and maintenance of outpatient anaesthesia with a propofol-volatile anaesthetic combination

Reference	Propofol administration [+]	Comparative maintenance	Principal findings[*]
Herregods et al., 1988	FRI	Isoflurane	Similar emergence and psychomotor performance
Larsen et al., 1992	FRI	Isoflurane	Impaired psychomotor performance for 30 min
Marshall et al., 1992	FRI	Isoflurane	Similar emergence and psychomotor performance
Milligan et al., 1987	IB	Isoflurane	Faster emergence, recovery times similar
Nightingale & Lewis, 1992	IB	Isoflurane	Improved psychomotor performance
Valanne, 1992	VRI	Isoflurane	Faster emergence, recovery, and discharge
Zuurmond et al., 1987	FRI	Isoflurane	Similar emergence and psychomotor performance
Ding et al., 1993	VRI	Enflurane	Similar emergence, recovery, and discharge
Rapp et al., 1992	VRI	Desflurane	Similar emergence and psychomotor performance
Van Hemelrijck et al., 1991	VRI	Desflurane	Similar emergence and psychomotor performance
Eriksson & Korttila, 1996	FRI	Desflurane	Similar emergence and psychomotor performance
Fredman et al., 1995	VRI	Sevoflurane	Similar emergence, recovery, and discharge

[+] VRI Variable rate infusion; FRI Fixed rate infusion; IB Intermittent bolus doses
[*] Findings are expressed with respect to the propofol group
Modified with permission from [14]

incidence of nocturnal oxygen desaturation during the first three post-operative days or in an earlier return of gastrointestinal function, improved mobility or reduced hospital stay, however[12]. In day case patients, propofol may reduce the hospital stay by virtue of its effects on PONV. In comparison to isoflurane, average discharge times were reduced from 235 ± 90 to 197 ± 55 min by the use of a propofol infusion.[11] Nausea particularly delayed discharge; average discharge time in patients with PONV was 267 ± 95 min compared to 185 ± 47 min in patients without PONV. In addition to a longer hospital stay, PONV also requires extra nursing and medical time, as well as additional drugs and supplies. The average cost per patient experiencing PONV has been estimated at US $15. Patients intensely dislike PONV and may even be willing to trade greater pain for less nausea. In addition to its unpleasantness and effect on the discharge time of day cases, PONV may also be associated with pulmonary aspiration, wound herniation, bleeding and rupture, and increased intra-ocular and intracranial pressure.

Propofol is now known to possess direct antiemetic properties and so the incidence of PONV will not necessarily be reduced with other iv anaesthetics. Etomidate is associated with a high incidence of PONV, as are all the opioid analgesics. The nausea associated with opioid analgesia has increased interest in alternative forms of pain relief, including concomitant use of local anaesthesia and the NSAIDs. Nevertheless, there is a definite need for a potent analgesic which does not cause nausea.

Other outcome measures

There is considerable debate about the effect of anaesthetic technique on a variety of outcome measures. Because of the difficulties already mentioned in performing these long term followup studies, most work has concentrated on major organ system function.

Cardiovascular disease is common with a high morbidity and mortality. When evaluating the incidence of postoperative CVS dysfunction, this must be related to the likelihood of developing similar problems in the absence of surgical intervention. As factors causing cardiovascular disease (e.g. smoking) may also increase the need for operations, it is difficult to evaluate the effect of surgery/anaesthesia in isolation.

Many studies comparing intravenous or volatile agents in patients with cardiovascular disease have failed to demonstrate major differences in cardiovascular outcome. Perioperative ischaemia is probably the most important factor in determining long term cardiac outcome. The provision of intense and effective analgesia with sufentanil (1 μg/kg/h) resulted in fewer and less severe ischaemic episodes in the intensive care unit following cardiac bypass compared to patients who received intermittent morphine for analgesia.[13] These differences in ischaemia only lasted during the period of intense analgesia and did not change short-term outcome endpoints such as reinfarction[13]. Similarly, other workers have shown that effective intraoperative analgesia can reduce postoperative myocardial ischaemia, although the long term implications of this are unknown.

In contrast to cardiovascular morbidity, postoperative pulmonary function appears to be worse in association with the use of opioid analgesics, consistent with their known respiratory depressant effects. Other aspects of the anaesthetic technique (e.g. volatile anaesthetic versus iv hypnotics) appear to have minimal effect, however.

Although postoperative neurological deficit is common after neurosurgical and cardiac procedures, no anaesthetic technique has consistently been shown to reduce this problem compared to the available alternatives. In a variety of animal models of neurological ischaemia, the barbiturates have been demonstrated to have a neuroprotective effect. This benefit has not been observed consistently in clinical practice, however.

Animal and *in vitro* studies have also shown a greater effect of volatile anaesthetics on immune function compared to iv anaesthetic agents. While these effects could theoretically affect both postoperative infection rates and tumour proliferation, no clinically significant differences have been detected in practice.

Summary

There are both advantages and disadvantages associated with intravenous anaesthesia. Intravenous anaesthesia usually requires the administration of several different substances to produce a complete anaesthetic, but using iv drugs in combination frequently results in interactions. These interactions may be beneficial in producing a greater (or more consistent) effect, as well as in reducing drug costs. Interactions may result in an enhanced desired effect while reducing the toxicity associated with the use of a larger dose of a single agent. Interactions may also result in enhanced toxicity, however, and the practitioner should always take care when using more than one drug, in case unexpected effects should occur.

Toxicity is an important concern with any form of drug therapy. There are a few uncommon but well recognised forms of toxicity associated with inhaled anaesthetics. These include malignant hyperpyrexia and "halothane" hepatitis. These conditions can be avoided by the use of iv anaesthetics. In most other patients, the various potential problems with the inhaled anaesthetics are more theoretical than real and overall outcome appears to differ little between iv and inhalational anaesthesia. In the presence of other diseases, the balance of risks and benefits may be altered and assessment of each individual patient is important.

Assessment of long term postanaesthetic outcome is difficult. Small differences in immediate recovery are relatively easy to demonstrate between different anaesthetic techniques. With improvements in both iv and volatile anaesthetics, these differences are becoming increasingly smaller, however. It is tempting to speculate that more rapid awakening will be associated with reduced costs and/or improved patient wellbeing. In practice, costs are dependent on many factors, while differences in long term outcome are difficult to demonstrate. Improvements in PONV are often observed with TIVA, but only when propofol is used. Furthermore, PONV is multifactorial and is especially influenced by the use of opioid analgesics. Other long term effects of anaesthetic technique on outcome have rarely been shown. Anaesthesia is becoming increasingly safe with favourable postoperative outcome. It is likely that careful, well controlled anaesthesia which avoids or minimises perioperative ischaemia is more important in determining outcome than the specific anaesthetic and analgesic agents used.

1 Smith I, Nathanson M, White PF. Sevoflurane – a long-awaited volatile anaesthetic. *Br J Anaesth* 1996;**76**:435–45.
2 Loewe S, Aldou RA, Fox SR, Johnson DG, Perkins W. Isobols of dose-effect relations in the combination of trimethadione and pentylenetetrazole. *J Pharmacol Exp Ther* 1955;**113**:475–80.
3 Bailey PL, Pace NL, Ashburn MA, *et al*. Frequent hypoxemia and apnea after sedation with midazolam and fentanyl. *Anesthesiology* 1990;**73**:826–30.
4 Halford FJ. A critique of intravenous anesthesia in war surgery. *Anesthesiology* 1943;**4**:67–9.
5 Cohen MM, Duncan PG, Pope WDB, Wolkenstein C. A survey of 112,000 anaesthetics at one teaching hospital (1975–83). *Can Anaesth Soc J* 1986;**33**:22–31.
6 Jellish WS, Lien CA, Fontenot HJ, Hall R. The comparative effects of sevoflurane versus propofol in the inductions and maintenance of anesthesia in adult patients. *Anesth Analg* 1996;**82**:479–85.
7 Van Hemelrijck J, Smith I, White PF. Use of desflurane for outpatient anesthesia: a comparison with propofol and nitrous oxide. *Anesthesiology* 1991;**75**:197–203.
8 Sung YF, Reiss N, Tillette T. The differential cost of anesthesia and recovery with propofol-nitrous oxide anesthesia versus thiopental sodium-nitrous oxide anesthesia. *J Clin Anesth* 1991;**3**:391–4.
9 Pollard BJ, Bryan A, Bennett D, *et al*. Recovery after oral surgery with halothane, enflurane, isoflurane or propofol anaesthesia. *Br J Anaesth* 1994;**72**:559–66.
10 Kalman SH, Jensen AG, Ekberg K, Eintrei C. Early and late recovery after major abdominal surgery. Comparison between propofol anaesthesia with and without nitrous oxide and isoflurane anaesthesia. *Acta Anaesthesiol Scand* 1993;**37**:730–6.
11 Green G, Jonsson L. Nausea: the most important factor determining length of stay after ambulatory anaesthesia. A comparative study of isoflurane and/or propofol techniques. *Acta Anaesthesiol Scand* 1993;**37**:742–6.
12 Phillips AS, Mirakhur RK, Glen JB, Hunter SC. Total intravenous anaesthesia with propofol or inhalational anaesthesia with isoflurane for major abdominal surgery. *Anaesthesia* 1996;**51**:1055–9.
13 Mangano DT. Postoperative myocardial ischemia. Therapeutic trials using intensive analgesia following surgery. *Anesthesiology* 1992;**76**:342–53.
14 Smith I, White PF, Nathanson M, Gouldson R. Propofol: an update on its clinical use. *Anesthesiology* 1994;**81**:1005–43.

7: The future of intravenous anaesthesia

The practice of iv anaesthesia has evolved considerably since its inception. Considerable developments have occurred in the last few years with the preparation of more specific drugs with shorter durations of effect and reduced side effects. Our understanding of the pharmacology of iv anaesthetics has improved considerably, especially in the area of pharmacokinetics. As a consequence, we are better able to predict the response to iv drugs under a variety of circumstances and to anticipate the rate of recovery when these agents are administered for varying periods of time. Further developments and refinements in our knowledge of pharmacokinetics seem likely in the future, allowing even more precise drug administration in all individuals, irrespective of body composition and/or preexisting disease states.

Although we still have very little understanding of the basic mechanism of action of anaesthetic drugs, we are likely to develop more specific and precisely targeted hypnotics in the future. There is a clear need for an iv anaesthetic which does not cause cardiovascular depression or apnoea. Other drugs used for iv anaesthesia have more clearly understood actions (e.g. opioid analgesics, muscle relaxants) and it is therefore easier to produce highly specific drugs. While a range of exceedingly "clean" muscle relaxants are now available, there is still a need for a potent analgesic devoid of respiratory depression, nausea and vomiting, and other gastrointestinal side effects.

Short duration of action is a desirable property in iv anaesthetics, as this facilitates control of the anaesthetic state and also permits rapid recovery, even after prolonged anaesthesia. The availability of ester metabolised drugs (e.g. esmolol, remifentanil) allows a very brief duration of effect, apparently unaffected by duration of drug delivery and independent of major organ function and disease states. It is possible that similar chemical linkages could be incorporated into other classes of drugs used in iv anaesthesia (e.g. hypnotics, sedatives, muscle relaxants), providing a comprehensive range of short duration drugs for TIVA. When developing drugs which are extensively and rapidly metabolised, it is of course essential to ensure that the metabolites produced are neither pharmacologically active nor in any way toxic or harmful.

Unfortunately, the cost of new drug development is ever increasing while there is a concurrent drive to contain rising health care costs. For these reasons, it is likely that the development of truly new iv anaesthetics will be less rapid than in the past. Modification to existing drugs is possible, however, resulting in a reduction in side effects or more beneficial properties. Many commonly used iv anaesthetic drugs exist as a racemic mixture (e.g. thiopentone, ketamine, atracurium), while only one of the optical isomers may be responsible for the desired actions. Preparation of pure optical isomers is becoming more economical and may result in drugs with fewer side effects than at present. Although "optically pure" drugs will still have to undergo extensive clinical trials in order to satisfy the licensing authorities of their clinical effects and safety, this process will still be considerably less expensive than developing an entirely new compound.

Developments may also occur in the way in which iv drugs are delivered or directed after their administration. Several iv drugs can be delivered by inhalation, by absorption from the buccal, sublingual or nasal mucosa and transdermally, using either passive diffusion or iontophoresis. Although no longer strictly iv drugs, these alternative routes of administration may offer many of the benefits of current iv medications but in a less invasive form, possibly with fewer side effects. These non-invasive drug delivery means may be particularly useful for premedication and for postoperative analgesia. A variety of non-invasive "patient controlled" options are possible with these delivery systems. A number of new concepts in drug delivery are already commercially available (at least in some countries) including the fentanyl Oralette®, the fentanyl skin patch and a metered nasal spray with a "lockout" period for patient controlled analgesia using a variety of opioid analgesics. Other devices are at varying stages of development.

Focusing potent drugs towards their principal site of effect may reduce the amount of drug reaching peripheral sites and therefore prevent them from causing undesirable effects at these locations. Possible means for targeting drug administration include the use of external physical forces to direct the drug itself, drug encapsulated in microspheres, and the use of monoclonal antibodies (specific to parts of a receptor) attached to existing iv drugs.

It may in time become possible to measure the concentration of iv drugs in the plasma in real time, allowing modifications to be made to the rate of drug delivery, in order to maintain a constant, desired concentration. It is already known, however, that there is a relatively poor correlation between plasma drug concentration and effect between individuals, perhaps as the concentration in the plasma does not reflect that at the effect site. Development of a monitor of the anaesthetic effect would overcome this problem and provide a more reliable endpoint against which to titrate drug delivery. With such a monitor, automatic, closed loop feedback of anaesthetic administration would become possible. Promising developments have been made in this area in recent years, with parameters derived from the processed EEG[1, 2] and auditory evoked potentials[3] currently appearing the most useful indices of anaesthetic effect.

Intravenous anaesthesia offers several advantages over the volatile agents in a variety of circumstances. Improvements in drug specificity with fewer undesirable effects, as well as more rapid recovery and response to changes in delivered concentration, will increase these advantages in the future. As concerns about environmental pollution intensify and as levels of other ozone depleting chemicals are reduced, the significance of inhaled anaesthetics will become relatively greater. Intravenous anaesthesia overcomes this source of environmental pollution, although the effects of drug manufacture and of discarded plastic syringes and infusion tubing on the environment must not be discounted.

Developments in surgical technique have had a major impact on anaesthetic practice in the past, with changing needs associated with a move towards day case operations and minimally invasive techniques. Further developments in surgical technique may reduce the requirement for general anaesthesia, with more procedures being amenable to sedative techniques. The iv hypnotic and analgesic drugs are ideal for use as sedatives. If more effective yet highly specific analgesics can be developed, it may even be possible to perform more extensive operations painlessly on awake or lightly sedated patients.

Summary

Anaesthesia has only been in existence for 150 years, while effective iv anesthetic drugs have only been available for less than half that time. Many of the currently used iv anaesthetic and adjuvant drugs (e.g. propofol, midazolam, alfentanil) and techniques (e.g. TIVA, sedoanalgesia, patient controlled sedation) have only been available for less than two decades. Given the significant advances which have occurred in the last five years (e.g. target controlled drug delivery, EEG bispectral index monitor, remifentanil, mivacurium, rocuronium, ORG 9487), the future of intravenous anaesthesia should be exciting as we enter the 21st century.

1 Glass PSA, Bloom M, Kearse L, et al. Bispectral analysis measures sedation and memory effects of propofol, midazolam, isoflurane, and alfentanil in healthy volunteers. *Anesthesiology* 1997;**86**:836–47.
2 Sebel PS, Bowles SM, Saini V, Chamoun N. EEG bispectrum predicts movement during thiopental/isoflurane anesthesia. *J Clin Monit* 1995;**11**:83–91.
3 Thornton C, Konieczko KM, Knight AB, et al. Effect of propofol on the auditory evoked response and oesophageal contractility. *Br J Anaesth* 1989;**63**:411–7.

Index

Printed and bound by CPI Group (UK) Ltd, Croydon, CR0 4YY

27/10/2024

14580393-0001